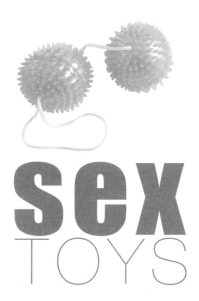

sex
TOYS

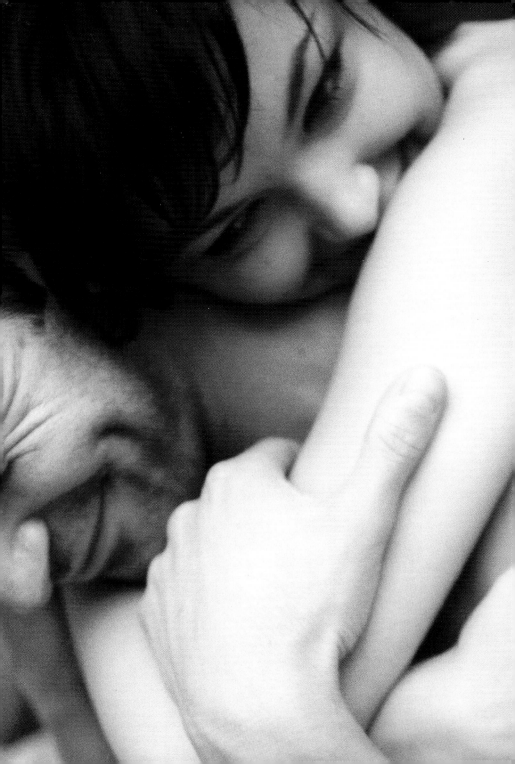

sex
TOYS

anne hooper

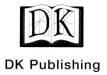

DK Publishing

First published in 2003 in the United Kingdom by:

Carroll & Brown Publishers Limited
20 Lonsdale Road
London NW6 6RD

Project Editor Ian Wood
Editor Stuart Moorhouse
Art Editor Luis Peral-Aranda
Photographer Jules Selmes
Photographic Assistant David Yems

First American Edition, 2003

00 01 02 03 04 05 10 9 8 7 6 5 4 3 2 1

Published in the United States by DK Publishing, Inc.
375 Hudson Street, New York, New York 10014

A Cataloging-in-Publication record for this book is available
from the Library of Congress ISBN 0-7894-9964-9

Reproduced by RALI
Printed and bound in Singapore by Tien Wah Press

Discover more at
www.dk.com

contents

bare essentials

From society's hypocritical attitudes to historical steam-powered dildos, here's everything you ever wanted to know about sex toys but were afraid to ask.

what's the big deal?

If we'd tried to produce a book on sex toys even 10 years ago, we would probably have failed. It's doubtful whether any mainstream bookstore would have stocked it, because public opinion then was that sex toys were "not quite nice."

But times have changed. Today's women see sexual playthings as a fun addition to the bedroom. Instead of treating their sex toys as a guilty secret to be hidden at the back of the closet, women are now more up-front and honest about them. They openly discuss the effects of vibrators and anal beads, and flock to erotic parties to buy the latest sex toys.

Vibrator usage is now so acceptable that I was recently consulted by a medical equipment company whose brief is to design a vibrator for use by women with sex problems. We might even be talking soon about vibrators on prescription. How times change!

the female market

Of course, women have received a little assistance in becoming so sexually open. Newspapers, women's magazines, and TV shows such as *Sex and the City* discuss sexual matters frankly, and the sex toy industry has woken up to women. After decades of ignoring their real needs, the sex toy manufacturers eventually realized they were missing out on half their sales potential. So they did something about it and adopted a more feminine approach to the design and color of their toys.

New materials—such as translucent rubber and latex that feels almost like real skin—paved the way for some very different sex toy designs. New technology has helped by making electrically operated toys more powerful and much quieter. Anyone who ever wrestled with the old-fashioned vibrator that shook, whirred, and resounded throughout the house will understand the advantages of silence.

buying sex toys

Many women dislike going into sex toy stores because most are still male-oriented, although there are many newer boutiques that are thoroughly woman-friendly. It is no accident that the most successful of these are often run by women. These include Good Vibrations in San Francisco, California, and the Ann Summers chain in the UK. There is also a growing number of women-only sex toy stores, the pioneer being the "Sh!" store in London, UK.

Women can also buy sex toys without embarrassment from virtual sex boutiques on the Internet. Both Good Vibrations and Ann Summers have their own websites, and there are many others. We list some of the best at the end of this book.

road-testing the toys

To help women (and their partners) learn more about sex toys, we decided to "road-test" the most popular models on the market. To do so, we recruited a small army of testers, both singles and couples. It wasn't difficult. We were swamped with applications. Our testers tried each toy and rated it for sexiness (how satisfying it was), noise-level, and value. We have summarized their comments and added extra information, such as tips on how to use the toys, similar products on the market, and the "According to Anne" sections, in which I give my own verdict on the products.

history of sex toys

Way back in the Stone Age, people began making tools from stones, bones, and antlers. These tools included hammers, axes, picks, and knives—and possibly dildos. In Europe in the 20th century, archaeologists discovered carved stone phalluses dating back to more than 12,000 years ago. Being archaeologists, they decided that these must be religious or symbolic items, despite the obvious fact that they were about the same size and shape as modern dildos, and one was even in the form of a double dildo.

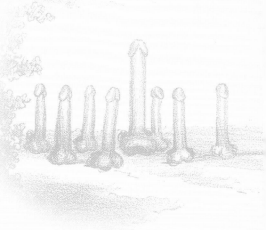

Sex toys aren't a new idea—like many things we think of as modern inventions, they've actually been around in one form or another for many thousands of years.

We'll never know for sure if Stone Age women used dildos, but it's very likely that women in Ancient Greece did. In Denmark, there's a Greek vase in Copenhagen's National Museum that shows a woman about to insert a long, slender dildo into her vagina while she raises a second one to her mouth. Other vases show figures holding small egg-shaped vessels, which held oil used for sexual lubrication. The Romans also made major use of dildos and manufactured them out of leather, bone, or wood. In the ancient city of Pompeii, now excavated from the lava that engulfed it many centuries ago, the murals in the brothel show some very interesting scenes.

medieval sex

In the 12th century, a European bishop reprimanded some of the women in his flock for "having made an instrument after the fashion of a male member, of a size to satisfy your desire, using this to commit fornication with other women, then using the same instrument on others as on yourself." Whoa!

The bishop's words seem to have had little effect, because the use of dildos continued throughout the following centuries. In the 1750s, for example, the Duchess of Tanis caused a huge scandal in Germany by getting herself married in male clothes to a girl to whom she made love using a dildo.

victorian delights

The Industrial Revolution brought technologies that eventually found uses in the budding sex toy industry of the Victorian era. With the advent of rubber, companies began making rubber dildos and clitoral stimulators. A French mail-order firm offered women a rubber sheath with soft points at the tip and a ridge on the head. This sheath fitted over the fingers, and the company also made double-ringed stimulators to be fitted over the penis.

The first vibrators appeared in 1869, when American physician George Taylor patented a steam-powered massage and vibratory apparatus. Unfortunately, the units were costly to make, difficult to move, and marketed for use by spas and physicians only. Up until around 1900, the use of vibrators was restricted to doctors, who used them to give women "medical massage" to relieve the symptoms of "hysteria." The first battery-operated vibrator was designed

Up until around 1900, the use of vibrators was restricted to doctors, who used them to give women "medical massage" to relieve the symptoms of "hysteria."

by British physician Joseph Mortimer Granville in 1880 and manufactured by the Weiss Company. By the turn of the century, more than a dozen manufacturers were producing both battery-powered vibrators and plug-in models.

modern times

Mail order was the standard way of selling vibrators and other sex toys in the first half of the 20th century, but retail sales through sex toy stores began to take off in the 1960s. Today, mail order, sex stores, and the Internet give easy access to the ever-growing range of sex toys on the market. The newest inventions include radio-controlled clitoral stimulators, electric galvanizers, and miniature finger vibrators made possible by new battery technology. In the near future, computer-controlled toys will be able to tailor their stimulation to meet their users' exact needs, and virtual reality toys will make our wildest fantasies feel like realities!

hitting the spot

Many types of sex toys, including vibrators, work best when you use them on the extra-sensitive regions of the body, which are called the erogenous zones. These parts of the body are rich in nerve endings that trigger intense sexual arousal when they are stimulated.

The first and absolutely basic rule about erogenous zones is that no two people are exactly alike. One partner's erogenous zones may be totally different to another's. So just because your last partner reacted explosively to having his or her nipples stroked, the same thing may leave your next lover cold.

To find your lover's erogenous zones, lightly stroke, lick, and kiss his or her whole body and note the reactions.

You can learn about your own erogenous zones by stroking them yourself, but it works much better if your lover does it for you. As you might expect, the genitals of both women and men are the prime erogenous zones.

the clitoris

For a woman, the clitoris is the powerhouse of sexual feeling. Although it responds readily to touch, it usually responds a great deal better when the rest of her body has been stroked and tenderly caressed. It is generally very difficult for a woman to climax without a lot of clitoral stimulation, but direct stimulation on the clitoris by a vibrator can sometimes be too intense. Many women react better to stimulation on the side of the clitoris.

a girl's erogenous zones can be

- Her ears and neck
- Her breasts and nipples
- The sides of her chest
- Her hands, wrists, and fingers
- The base of her abdomen
- Her clitoris
- The outside of her vagina (low sensation)
- Her G-spot

- Her perineum—the area between her vagina and her anus
- The outside rim of her anus
- Her buttocks
- The insides of her thighs
- The backs of her knees
- Her feet and toes

  Don't forget—not every girl will be the same.

the G-spot

Not every woman has one of these pleasure buttons, but if she does, it is located at the far end of the vagina on its upper wall. The G-spot is named after its discoverer, German gynecologist Ernst Grafenberg (1881–1957). It feels like a small, bean-sized bump, and responds erotically to sustained pressure. Some vibrators are made to pulsate instead of just vibrating, in order to deliver this pressure.

the penis

The most sensitive part of a man's penis is its head. It is usually covered by the foreskin, but not every guy turns up equipped with one of these. Many men are circumcized as babies for reasons of religion or hygiene. For intercourse and when using sex toy attachments, the foreskin needs to be rolled well back.

the prostate gland

Every man has one of these, located in front of the far end of the anus. It produces the seminal fluid that carries the sperm. As an erogenous zone, it is the man's equivalent of a woman's G-spot. Stimulating the prostate, by using a fingertip or anal probe to massage it through the front wall of the anus, results in easy and rapid orgasm.

a guy's erogenous zones can be

- His ears and neck
- His nipples
- The base of his abdomen
- His penis—especially its head
- His testicles
- His perineum—the area between the base of his penis and his anus
- The outside rim of his anus
- His prostate gland
- His buttocks
- The insides of his thighs
- The backs of his knees
- His feet and toes

Don't forget—not every guy will be the same.

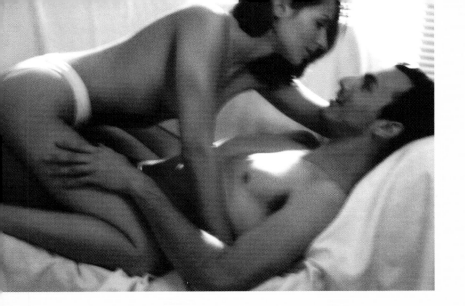

communication is the key

Does the following scenario sound familiar? You have bought a daring (for you) sex toy and you are longing to try it out with your partner. But so far your sex life—though joyous—has been just a little straightforward. Which is great, but you would love to introduce a little novelty into things. So, there you are with this neat little vibrator attachment for men (it fits onto the base of his penis) that promises to give you both extremely good vibes. But how on earth do you get him to wear it?

Among the thoughts that might be flying through your head is the awful possibility that he will be unpleasantly surprised. So much so that your present sex life will be irrevocably altered, for the worse. Other thoughts might include "Will he think I'm a slut (or a sex maniac) for suggesting this?" or "Will he think I'm suggesting that he's inadequate?"

If you find yourself in this predicament, the first thing to do is to make a serious assessment of your guy's temperament. If he really is the type to scream and run a mile when you suggest using a vibrator, say nothing and give the toy to one of your girlfriends.

But if you decide that he is probably up for it, you need to wipe away all the doubts, fears, and hesitations from your own mind. The key to using sex toys well is to be supremely confident about doing so. If you think sex toys are cool and really fun, then raising the subject in a direct manner will be both appropriate and natural. And he will take it in the manner in which it is given. If you hesitate and apologize, your partner might get the idea that there is something wrong with using sex toys. So be unashamed. You are entitled to your beliefs.

Anyway, most men react in pretty much the same way when asked how they might feel if their partners offered them special sexual treats. They don't exactly say that they'd think they'd died and gone to heaven, but they do look interested and entertained. At the very least, most men are open-minded enough to agree to experiment. The enthusiastic reactions of the men on the receiving end of our road-testing was proof of this.

so how do you start?

Begin by talking about your sex toy as you would about any other purchase. Don't make a big deal about it. Our testers found it helpful to go home and say "Guess what I've got to do for work, darling." Your line might be "Guess what I bought today." Some of our testers found themselves a little nervous after raising the subject like this. But the nervousness disappeared if they followed through by being positive about how much they were looking forward to sexual experimentation. It also helped them if they made sure their bedroom was tidy, warm, sweet-smelling, and romantically lit, with candles or one carefully shaded lamp.

Once in bed, getting started was easy. The sex-toy testers and their partners read the instructions together and then adapted their lovemaking to include using the toy. For example, if the toy was a vibrator they would make love in much the same way as usual, but had used the vibrator during foreplay for increased arousal.

using toys together

Good communication with your partner is as important when you use a sex toy as it is when you first suggest it. Here are some useful tips to help you get the most from a new toy:

When you are using the toy on your partner, ask regularly how it feels.

Listen to their reply and modify your moves accordingly.

When you are on the receiving end, give feedback without being asked. Say things like "Ooh, that feels wonderful," or "That's cool, but it would be even better lower down." Never say "That's terrible." Always encourage your partner by showing appreciation, then going on to suggest ways that would improve the experience for you.

Give each other time. Climaxes are almost always better when you have been building up sexual excitement.

Always remember the value of moaning with delight! It really lets your partner know that he or she is doing something right.

sexy edibles | inside secrets | fun and games

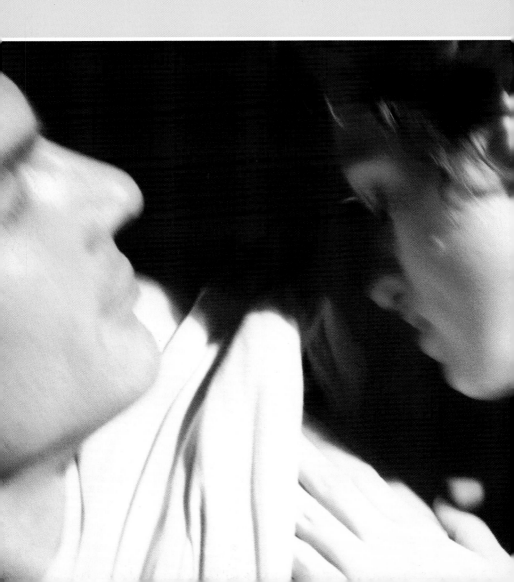

toys to
toy with

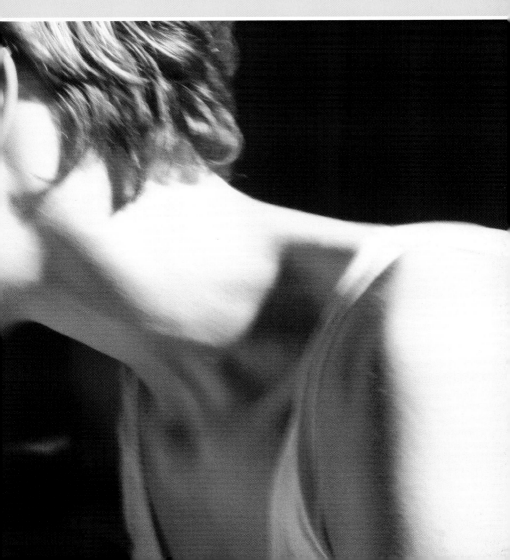

sexy edibles

Would you rather make love or dive into a box of chocolates? Difficult decision? Then why not combine the two? Satisfy more than just your sexual appetite by introducing these tasty treats into your bedroom activities.

Sexy edibles are great to both get you in the mood for love and as a teasing temptation during foreplay. Why eat food from a spoon when you could be enjoying it in *far* more interesting ways? If you are in a long-term relationship, these sexy edibles can work wonders in bringing an element of surprise back into your sex life.

ginger. These guarantee added sensual pleasure for both you and your partner. And once you find a flavor you like, you won't want to stop!

lickable lingerie

Edible underwear for both men and women is now widely available. So, surprise your partner by greeting him or

> "Great food is like great sex—the more you have the more you want."
>
> GAEL GREENE

naughty sauces

If you want to add more flavor to your oral lovemaking, you can rub on a range of tasty edible gels and creams in flavors such as mint, strawberry, passion fruit, and cinnamon before you start. Be sure to note that these are suitable for use only on external skin. Otherwise—ouch! Also available are edible massage oils in flavors such as hazlenut, lime, and

her at the door in nothing but some sexy underwear. He or she will be even more surprised to discover that no hands are needed to remove it. You can buy beautiful panties and bras made of rice paper decorated with sugar, or you can go for a different effect with gummy undies that dissolve when your lover licks, nibbles, or sucks them. It all depends on what tickles your tastebuds.

edible body art

You can use body paints in all sorts of sexy and fun ways—just let your artistic imagination run free!

painting yourself
Paint the parts of your body that your partner loves most as a delicious surprise for him or her to savor. Or use the paint to write suggestive words and naughty pictures that reveal your desires.

painting your partner
Paint the parts of your partner's body that you love most, then lick the paint off with long, slow strokes of your tongue. Paint saucy sentences or shapes on your partner's body, then before you lick them off, ask him or her to guess what they are.

consumable cuffs
If you're feeling particularly adventurous, what about the extra excitement of letting your partner tie you up while he or she "undresses" you? You can Indulge in all the fantasy but none of the dangers of bondage by using edible handcuffs. Try eating your way to freedom or let your partner "rescue" you—or take advantage of your helplessness!

provocative paints
Spoil yourself, and get artistic, with some silky-smooth body paint. It's great fun to apply and even more fun to remove. Catering to all tastes, these body paints are available in milk, dark, or white chocolate, as well as a range of fruit flavors. Most come complete with brushes, but you can use your fingers if you prefer—just rub on and lick off. As an alternative, try flavored edible body powder. Slowly brush it onto your partner with a soft brush or a feather, then lick it off.

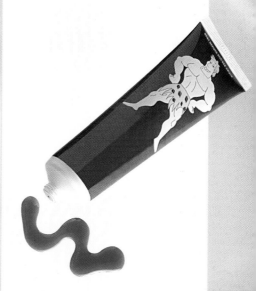

edible undies

Chew your way to heaven with these erotic novelties that bring flavor to foreplay. Edible undies don't offer a great taste sensation and you probably wouldn't want to eat a whole one, but you can have fun trying.

Edible panties

minimalist | gummy | strawberry chocolate

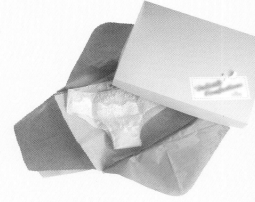

Mike's test drive

"These were great fun. The giggling started when we took them out of the box, they were so tiny and dainty! My partner had to be careful putting them on for fear of tearing them, and they revealed more than they covered (no bad thing). I started off by licking them, but as they warmed up they started to melt and get sticky. So I used my lips to pull them away from my partner's body and then chewed them. There wasn't much flavor, and when they stuck to my teeth and stained my mouth red we were soon both laughing too much to carry on. So I just pulled them off her and we made happy, giggly love."

sexiness: *sassy*
value: *cheap for the price*

according to ANNE

Taking your lover's underwear off with your teeth is a classic sex move that everyone should have perfected. These edible undies let you take it further and really make a meal out of your dental undressing!

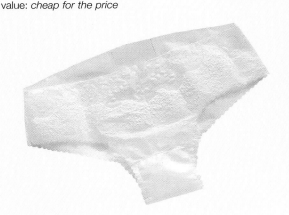

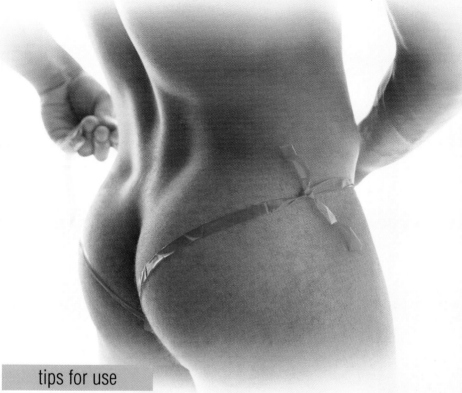

tips for use

Start off by licking the undies to soften them, and be careful not to give your partner a painful bite when you're chewing into the material. You have to work quite quickly, otherwise your partner's body heat will melt the undies and make them stick to his or her body and pubic hairs. But don't just rip them off with your teeth— much of the fun lies in gradually nibbling away at them, even though it can be messy.

Men's briefs

one size (almost) fits all | gummy | cherry

Sarah's test drive

"These were more like bikini bottoms than men's briefs—just a triangle of flimsy gum tied at the hip with thin gummy ribbons. When I started licking at them, they softened and my aroused partner started to burst out of them. As I nibbled away at them (and him), they started to break up and stick to his pubic hairs, and I had to snuffle around in his crotch to get at the gooey little blobs of cherry-flavored gloop. We both found this very funny, but all the licking and sucking soon got him quite worked up and hungry for sex. I think this would be a good way to get your man in the mood if his enthusiasm was ever less than total."

sexiness: *throbbing*
value: *cheap and cheerful*

the lick of love

Try exploring your erotic creativity with edible body paints and powders, or indulge in the sweet, sensual pleasures of sexy candies that will help you and your partner get in the mood for love.

Honey Dust
3.5 oz (100g) | honey flavor

Marilyn's test drive
"This is like a sweet-tasting talcum powder. I enjoyed dusting it onto myself with the feather applicator, and enjoyed it even more when my partner did it for me. He loved the smell and taste of it on my skin, and he spent ages kissing and licking me all over. That was a real bonus, as foreplay isn't usually his strong point!"

sexiness: *sizzling*
value: *worth its weight in gold*

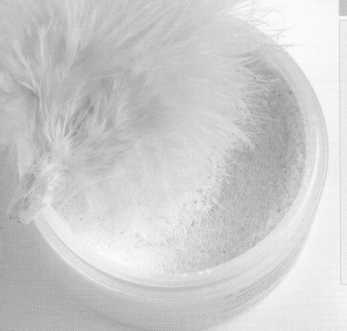

according to ANNE

You don't always need body paints or powders to have sexy edible fun. Try spreading your lover's body with sticky honey or thick, silky cream, or an ordinary chocolate or nut spread. Then treat your lover to the sweet sensation of your lapping tongue on their eager skin!

tips for use

sexy candy

Certain foods can be sensual in their own right, while others are associated with the thought of sexuality. Suggestively shaped candies, especially chocolates, combine both these features. Chocolate contains phenylethylamine (PEA), a chemical that stimulates and enhances the senses. Nibble some together before you go to bed, to get yourselves in a warm, sexy mood.

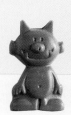 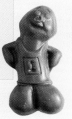

spoilt for choice

CHOCOLATE BITS: cute little chocolate shapes—including naughty nobs, delicious nipples, and sassy demons.

EDIBLE HANDCUFFS: try a little sweet bondage with handcuffs made of chocolate or of fruit-flavored gum.

CANDY WHIP: whip up some passion with a gummy whip, then eat it to destroy the evidence!

PENIS PASTA: penis-shaped pasta—best eaten al dente with a spicy sauce! Also available in boob shapes.

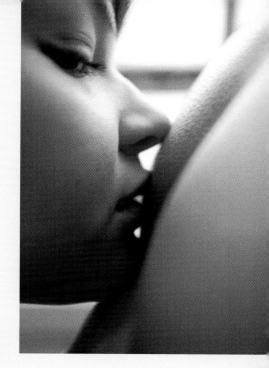

Chocolate Body Paint

5.3 oz (150 g) tube | mint chocolate | applicator

Steve's test drive

"This paint comes in a tube, (like a toothpaste tube), and includes a brush to paint it on with. As it's a bit runny when it comes out of the tube, we were glad my partner had thought to spread out an old towel to lie on before we started using it. To try it out, I began by painting her nipples. Once the paint was on, it dried quickly and we both enjoyed me licking it off again. It tasted great. Then we took turns at painting each other, but without the brush. It was more fun just drizzling the paint straight from the tube. We both loved playing with this paint, and we're looking forward to trying out other flavors."

sexiness: *saucy*
value: *an economical delicacy*

inside secrets

Tiny sex toys that you can tuck away inside you, or wear under your clothing, will give you deliciously hot, hands-free pleasure. Some are so small and silent that you can even use them in public and no one will ever guess your sinful secret!

The latest miniature sex toys vary from metal balls that slip inside your vagina, to little remote-controlled vibrators about the size of your thumb. Many women find them easier to use than larger toys, and they often appeal to sex-toy rookies who feel a little intimidated by the full-sized models. For the lowdown on these fun-sized joy-toys—read on!

forward as if you were making love. Use them for solo pleasuring or extra sensations during lovemaking.

If you want a more intense experience, you could try love balls covered with soft latex spikes, or experiment with the battery-powered vibrating versions.

> "A secret is not something unrevealed, but something told privately, in a whisper."
> MARCEL PAGNOL

love balls
The simplest types of love balls, a.k.a. Chinese balls or love eggs, are pairs of smooth metal or weighted plastic balls that nestle inside your vagina. As you move around, they shift position and gently stimulate you. Of course, how you move is up to you! For an extra-sexy sensation, gently rock your pelvis from side to side, or thrust it backward and

vibrating panties
This novel form of personal pleasuring is basically a pair of skimpy panties with a pocket holding a small vibrator that presses against your clitoris. These can be great fun, but some women find that they don't fit tightly enough to hold the vibrator sufficiently in place—wearing pantyhose over them can often increase the pressure.

tips for use

squeeze for success
Want better orgasms? Then try using love balls to tone up your PC (pubococcygeal) muscles. These muscles support your pelvic floor, and they contract rhythmically during orgasm. Strong PC muscles will give you a tighter vagina and more powerful orgasms. You can strengthen your PC muscles by using a simple exercise, that can be made even more effective by putting love balls inside your vagina to give it something to squeeze against.

PC workout
To find your PC muscles, practice stopping the flow of urine when you take a pee—the muscles you use to do this are your PC muscles. To strengthen them, contract them for three seconds, relax them for three seconds, then contract them again. Do this ten times, three times a day. To check on your progress, lie down and slip a finger into your vagina, then see how tightly you can squeeze it with your PC muscles.

If that doesn't do the trick, you can use the vibrator with ordinary panties that don't have the gusset sewn up at both sides—just slip the vibrator into the gusset!

remote-controlled vibrators
These little bullet-shaped vibrators have their batteries in a separate power pack that doubles as a remote-control unit. Slip one into your vagina, switch on, and enjoy the buzz!

Most of these little pleasure packs have more than one speed setting, so you can vary the intensity of the effect. You can also use them on your clitoris and your nipples—or let your partner operate the remote control to tease you with unexpected speed changes!

great balls of love

These "ecstasy balls" slip inside your vagina for solo enjoyment or for extra stimulation during intercourse. They may be small, but they'll put a big smile on your face!

Ben Wa Gold Balls

0.7 inch (1.8 cm) diameter | metal | non-vibrating | crystal-look case

Stella's test drive

"These balls are quite small, so I could hardly feel them when I first popped them in. But I soon discovered that rocking backward and forward gave me subtle, sexy sensations, and some gentle pelvic thrusting made this even better. Despite the occasional sound of metal against metal, I completely relaxed into the experience, and even ended up enjoying the exploration to remove the balls. Next time, I'll insert my finger for longer while the Ben Wa balls are inside me, or I'll use them with a partner during sex, to see if they help me to reach orgasm. I'm looking forward to it already!"

sexiness: *filling* value: *bargain*
sound effect: *clinky*

according to ANNE

Once you are comfortable wearing the silent variety around the house, why not wear them outside? They could be just the thing to spice up a routine shopping trip or a dull morning at the office. Just bear in mind that you should only leave them in for a few hours at a time.

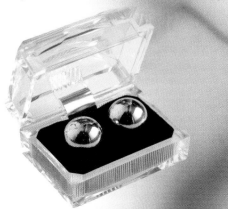

Vibrating Luv Balls

1.4 inch (3.6 cm) diameter | Ultra Skin coated |
separate battery pack | twisting speed adjuster

Jenny's test drive

"I got a huge kick out of having two balls
entirely inside me and I was particularly turned
on by their soft texture, which really felt like
skin inside me. I loved the feeling of being in
complete control of the vibration intensity I
received. It was also great that I could just
gently pull the cord to remove them."

sexiness: *subtle* value: *worth every cent*
sound effect: *chatterbox*

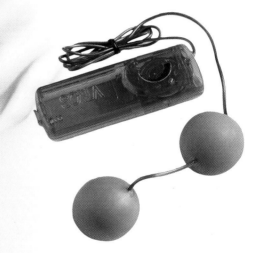

Textured Duo Balls

1.5 inch (3.8 cm) diameter | latex-covered metal |
non-vibrating | soft but spiky texture

Maureen's test drive

"The girlie pink of these balls held instant sex
appeal for me. Then the feel of the soft spikes
inside me drove me wild: tickly in some places
and entirely orgasmic in others! I also
experimented by tugging lightly on the cord
now and again to move the balls around a bit,
which made it feel better still. Wow!"

sexiness: *spiky, but nice*
value: *cheap for the price*

some secret treats

This selection of intimate toys—each a "secret" in its own unique way—shows only a few of the many delightful alternatives to traditional vibrators that are on offer for women to amuse themselves with in private.

Tiger panties

G-string sized | leopardskin-print Lycra | attached battery pack | adjustable speed

Alice's test drive

"The mere thought of these filled me with excitement, I think because of the idea of having naughty secrets in public! I put on the panties in my bedroom to try them out, switched on the tiny vibrator, and slipped it into the discreet front pocket, rubbing it on my clit on the way. But the pants were too big for me, so the bullet wasn't tight enough to my clitoris for me to feel much vibration. The sensation was much better when I pressed the panties firmly against myself, but I think I might look a little odd if I ever did this in public! I would like to try a tighter pair so that the bullet could sit firmly on my clitoris. And a pair that didn't buzz quite so conspicuously would give an increased element of secrecy and surprise!"

sexiness: *flips your switch* value: *hard on the pocket*
sound effect: *fortissimo*

according to ANNE

The remote-controlled bullet vibrators may be small but they still pack quite a punch. And because you can leave them comfortably inside your vagina without having to hold them in place, they leave your hands free to explore and caress your own body—or your partner's!

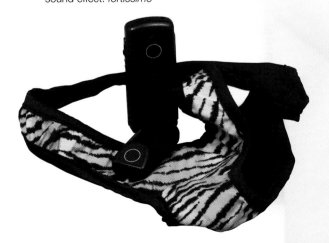

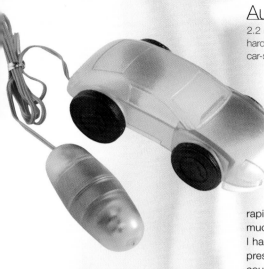

Auto Erotica

2.2 inches (5.6 cm) long x 0.8 inches (2 cm) wide | hard plastic | batteries within the car | car-shaped controller

Kiara's test drive

"I found this pink car-shaped toy funny, but also very sexy. The fact that the wheels were the on/off switches and speed adjusters and that you open the trunk to put in the batteries gave me a real buzz. First I held it against my clit and then started circling around it. In its most rapid mode the Auto Erotica was almost too much for me, and because of the hard texture I had to be careful not to apply too much pressure. I'd recommend this toy to anyone—I couldn't get enough!"

sexiness: *gets your heart racing*
value: *it's a steal*
sound effect: *purrs*

EZ Pleaser

2.5 inches (6 cm) long | jelly sleeve | separate battery pack | adjustable speed

Harriet's test drive

"The modern silver bullet, the feminine pink sleeve, and the unintimidating size were the initial attractions of this toy. The bullet provided exhilarating sensations on my nipples and inner thighs, but when I used it on my 'special place' I preferred the feel of the knobbly sleeve against me. My partner got really turned on by remote-teasing me, but then I grabbed it off him and used it briefly inside me, along with his finger, to climax. This toy is great for use with a boyfriend, as well as being ideal for solo ventures."

sexiness: *dead sexy* value: *worth every cent*
sound effect: *talkative*

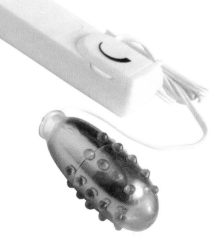

fun and games

If you like games and you like sex, why not combine the two? From kinky card games to dressing up in outrageous outfits, playing sexy games is the perfect way to spice up your evenings in!

Sex games have been part of humanity's sexual repertoire for thousands of years. Ancient sex manuals such as the *Kama Sutra* often recommend their use during both courtship and foreplay. When you and your partner play sexy games, you enjoy a shared experience that brings you closer, makes you laugh, and breaks down inhibitions. It also turns you on…

the loser an item of clothing. For fairness, just make sure you're both wearing the same number of clothes before you start!

contact sports

Your skin is more than just a waterproof covering that helps keep your body parts in place. It's your body's biggest

> "Give a man a free hand and he'll run it all over you."
> MAE WEST

games people play

Most sex toy stores now stock a range of erotic card and board games. Some of them create sexy mental fun to stir your libido. Others take a more hands-on approach by accentuating the physical to add fun to foreplay.
If none of the commercial games appeals to you, there's always the old standby of strip poker—all you need is an ordinary pack of cards. And if neither of you know the rules of poker (it can happen!) you can substitute any other card game where a bum hand can cost

single organ and, thanks to its millions of highly sensitive nerve endings, it's also your biggest sex organ. That's why touching and being touched is the key to good foreplay, whether the touch is light and playful or slow and sensual. The gentle, teasing touch of soft materials such as silk, feathers, and fur can generate a powerful erotic charge. Get your partner to trail a soft feather or a silk scarf along your naked body. It will make you tingle with lust—especially if you wear a blindfold to heighten your sensitivity to touch.

erotic massage strokes

To give a truly erotic massage, first prepare the scene by making sure the room is warm and softly lit. Spread out towels or an old (but clean) sheet for your partner to lie on, because massage oils can stain. Warm the oil by standing the bottle in a bowl of warm water, then gently rub some of it onto your hands.

When you give the massage, use sexy strokes like these:

- trace the outline of your partner's ears with your fingertips

- breathe softly into the ears and onto the neck

- gently knead the muscles between the shoulderblades and at the base of the neck

- glide your fingernails down the inside of each arm

- circle the nipples with your fingernails

- gently squeeze the nipples between fingers and thumbs

- stroke the sides of the breasts and breathe on the nipples

- move your palms in circles on your partner's buttocks

- firmly squeeze and knead each buttock in turn

- run your fingertips lightly up the inside of each thigh...

For a more intimate and romantic tactile experience, give each other a sensual massage. Make it a long, languorous, and erotic experience, aimed at arousing the senses. You can massage with dry hands, but your movements will be smoother and sexier if you rub some massage oil onto your fingers and palms. Massage oils are lighter and less greasy than baby oil, and many contain essential oils such as sandalwood, jasmine, and rose.

To enhance the skin-tingling effect, use a latex massage mitt with a textured surface, or a soft and sensuous fur mitt. But never use massage oil with a fur (or fake fur) mitt—it'll soon have the look and feel of an old wet dog.

dress to thrill

Raise your lover's lust-level with sensuous, provocative lingerie that tempts and teases, or add some fun to your bedroom frolics with a sexy uniform or a fantasy costume.

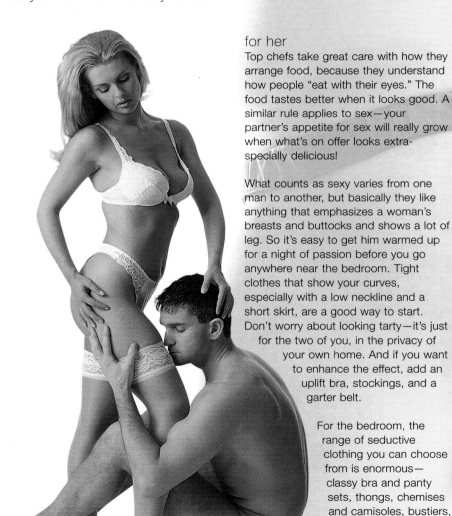

for her

Top chefs take great care with how they arrange food, because they understand how people "eat with their eyes." The food tastes better when it looks good. A similar rule applies to sex—your partner's appetite for sex will really grow when what's on offer looks extra-specially delicious!

What counts as sexy varies from one man to another, but basically they like anything that emphasizes a woman's breasts and buttocks and shows a lot of leg. So it's easy to get him warmed up for a night of passion before you go anywhere near the bedroom. Tight clothes that show your curves, especially with a low neckline and a short skirt, are a good way to start. Don't worry about looking tarty—it's just for the two of you, in the privacy of your own home. And if you want to enhance the effect, add an uplift bra, stockings, and a garter belt.

For the bedroom, the range of seductive clothing you can choose from is enormous—classy bra and panty sets, thongs, chemises and camisoles, bustiers, basques, and also

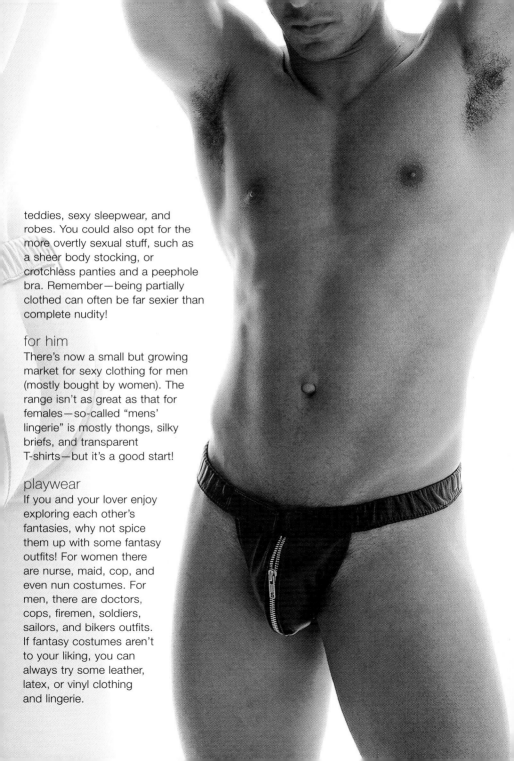

teddies, sexy sleepwear, and robes. You could also opt for the more overtly sexual stuff, such as a sheer body stocking, or crotchless panties and a peephole bra. Remember—being partially clothed can often be far sexier than complete nudity!

for him

There's now a small but growing market for sexy clothing for men (mostly bought by women). The range isn't as great as that for females—so-called "mens' lingerie" is mostly thongs, silky briefs, and transparent T-shirts—but it's a good start!

playwear

If you and your lover enjoy exploring each other's fantasies, why not spice them up with some fantasy outfits! For women there are nurse, maid, cop, and even nun costumes. For men, there are doctors, cops, firemen, soldiers, sailors, and bikers outfits. If fantasy costumes aren't to your liking, you can always try some leather, latex, or vinyl clothing and lingerie.

card and board games

Spice up any card game with Booby Match, the breast game in town. Or improve your foreplay skills and indulge in some adventurous fantasy sex with Nookii or Monogamy.

Booby Match
card game | can be used as ordinary playing cards

Simon's test drive
"This is a great game. It's a pack of large playing cards with pictures of boobs on them. I particularly liked the presentation—the real puppies on the box and the large size of the cards. The idea is to sort the boobs into matching pairs, which sounds easy but was surprisingly difficult. I have to admit it turned me on: I'm not used to seeing so many boobs—of all shapes, sizes, and shades—in one evening. I soon had particular favorites among them. Forget any reservations about the cards being tacky or offensive. Just enjoy them for what they are—a bit of harmless fun."

sexiness: *heaving* value: *bargain*

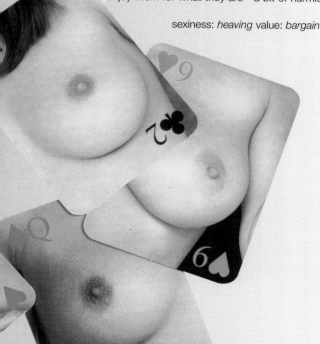

according to ANNE

Sexy game-playing is a fun way to pep up your sex life. With a new partner, it helps you get to know each other better by breaking down inhibitions. And when you're in an established relationship, it helps you keep your sex life as adventurous and exciting as it was at the beginning.

Nookii

dice and sexy activity card game | silk scarf for a blindfold

Maya's test drive

"This is like a grown-ups' version of the kids' game where they dare each other to do naughty things. The 'dares' come from the instructions on the cards, and they get you doing all sorts of sexy things to each other. You end up doing a sort of combined foreplay and fantasy play. It's all great fun and very sexy! But it is very expensive."

sexiness: *almost too hot to handle*
value: *pricy—but worth it*

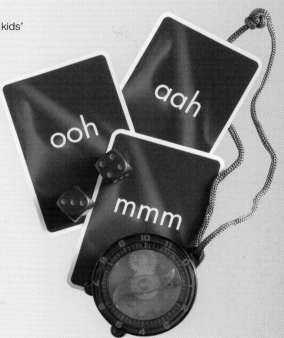

Monogamy

board game with question cards | fantasy cards

Heather's test drive

"The rules are easy to learn and remember, and you can choose from three different levels of questions about your most intimate thoughts and desires. This game's addictive, and we're both looking forward to acting out all the 50 different fantasies the winner gets to choose from at the end of each session."

sexiness: *sizzling*
value: *everyone's a winner*

gorgeous gifts

For a special occasion—or just because they're special—why not treat your lover to a sexy gift, such as a designer vibrator, some sumptuous silken sheets, or the poetic passions of an erotic novel.

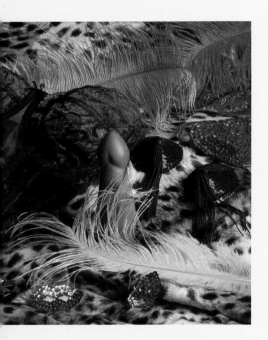

contraceptives with class

Luxury condoms: they're more than twice the price of most other condoms, but they are comfortable and sensitive and made of high-purity latex that cuts the risk of allergic reactions and is almost odorless. The attractive packaging looks good on the bedside table, too.

bedtime stories

Spark your lover's imagination with an erotic book. A good-quality edition of the *Kama Sutra* makes ideal bedtime reading, and there are illustrated editions for extra erotic inspiration. The *Kama Sutra*, while legendary for it's amazing range of sexual positions, also instructs on other aspects of the sexual experience, such as the importance of scent and color. You could also try works like the *Ananga Ranga* or *The Perfumed Garden.* If the style of the classics doesn't appeal, there's no shortage of modern guides to sex positions and sexual fantasies.

If your lover prefers erotica in story form, there's plenty to choose from. Erotic literature ranges from raunchy versions of romantic fiction to classier stuff such as Anaïs Nin's *Delta of Venus* and Pauline Reage's *The Story of O*, and novels such as those by Anne Rice under her pen-name A.N. Roquelaure.

designer vibes

If you're feeling extravagant, a designer vibe is a wonderful alternative to the usual phallic-shaped toys. Made of high-grade silicones and resins and fashioned into sensuously smooth and curvy shapes, these look more like small pieces of abstract sculpture than sex toys. They not only look great, they are also fully functioning multi-speed vibes, effective for both sexual stimulation and general body massage.

love packs

Most sex toy suppliers sell gift packs for both women and men. The packs for women usually include a vibe, lube, and toy cleaner, plus a small selection of other goodies, such as a clit stimulator or love balls. A typical men's pack might include a masturbation aid and a cock ring, plus lube and wipes. These packs make fun erotic gifts, and many of them are ideal starter kits for those new to the pleasure of sex toys.

sexy sheets

Add some luxury to your lovemaking by giving your partner some silk, satin, or even PVC bed sheets. These cool, slinky sheets are available in a range of sexy shades such as decadent gold, sinful scarlet, and wicked black.

massage magic

Lock the door, dim the lights, and get ready for some tactile treats. Tickle your lover's fancy with soft, sexy feathers, or stroke each other to ecstasy with a furry mitt or luxurious, seductively slippery massage oils.

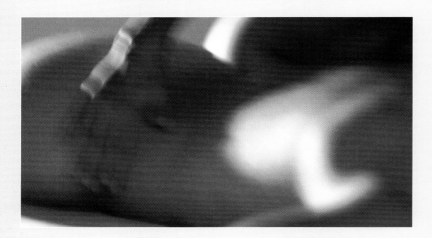

Massage oils
3-8 oz (30-237 ml) | vegetable oils

Vernon's test drive
"We always thought massage oils were just a gimmick, but we were pleasantly surprised at how effective they are. They make a massage much easier and sexier, and my partner really likes the way they make her skin feel softer and silkier. My favorites are the ones that gently heat up when you rub them in."

sexiness: *super-sensual*
value: *cheap for the price*

according to ANNE

Being tickled with feathers may not sound sexy but it can be truly sensational. Instead of feathers you could try a silk scarf, or if you have long hair you could sweep it slowly along your lover's body.

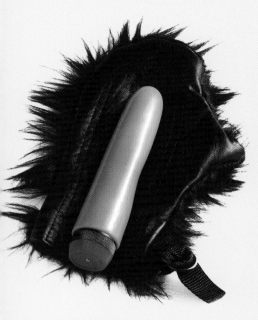

Furry Friend
one size fits all hands | fake fur

Harriet's test drive

"This massage mitt looks very odd—large and clumsy and somewhat like an animal's paw. But when my partner used it on me it actually felt quite nice, more warm and comforting than sexy, although not that sexy for my partner, who was getting very hot in the wrong way! When we slipped a slimline vibrator inside, it was really good fun, especially when he used in on my buttocks and the insides of my thighs!"

sexiness: *furry but fun*
value: *worth every cent*

Fantasy feathers
18 inches (46 cm) long | ostrich feather with plastic handle

Kay's test drive

"I surprised my boyfriend by coming into the bedroom wearing nothing but nail polish, with one of these long-handled feathers in each hand—strategically positioned to cover my 'private parts.' It was great fun to see the look of joy on his face. I asked him to lie down and climbed on top of him and started tickling him with the feathers, asking him where he most liked the sensation. I also wrote messages on his back with them, such as 'U R GR8,' to see if he could make them out by touch alone. He loved the feel of the feathers, and I did too when he used them on me! They are a very sexy addition to the bedroom—both as wicked toys and as great decorations."

sexiness: *exotically erotic*
value: *a complete bargain*

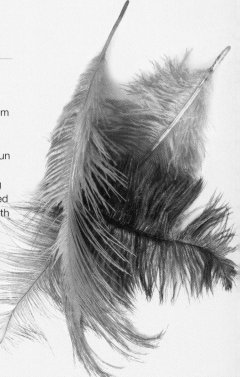

star sign vibrators

Match your pleasures to your personality with these velvety silicone vibes, which are styled to represent the essence of your astrological star sign.

Aries

A vibe to match the idealistic, romantic sign of Aries—shaped like a ram's head and colored a fiery red to fan the flames of passion.

Taurus

This contoured orange vibe is designed to please the strong, determined woman born under the sign of Taurus.

Gemini

A sunshine yellow vibe to appeal to the bright, versatile, but fickle nature of the Gemini woman.

Cancer

The sea-green color flecked with bubbles and crab motifs reflects the emotional depths of the woman born under the sign of Cancer.

Leo

A tawny-colored vibe that's sure to make the proud, playful Leo woman purr with pleasure.

Virgo

A light green vibe to loosen the inhibitions of the slightly shy but exceptionally sexy Virgo woman.

Libra

The elegant royal blue color of this vibe suits the charm of the romantic but contradictory Libran woman.

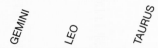

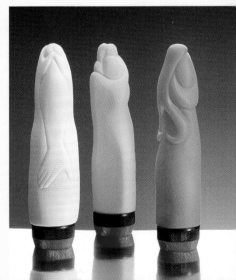

Scorpio

This scorpion-shaped vibe is colored deep red to match the intense, passionate nature of the Scorpio woman.

Sagittarius

Shaped like a rounded arrowhead to symbolize the adventurous sign of the Archer, this vibe is sure to hit its target.

Capricorn

The slick shape of this deep blue vibe makes it ideal for the polished, determined Capricorn woman.

Aquarius

With its flowing shape and Water Carrier motif, this vibe will help the imaginative Aquarian woman to float away on rippling streams of delight.

Pisces

Using this sleek, fish-shaped vibe, the sensitive Piscean woman can lie back and surrender to the waves of pleasure washing over her.

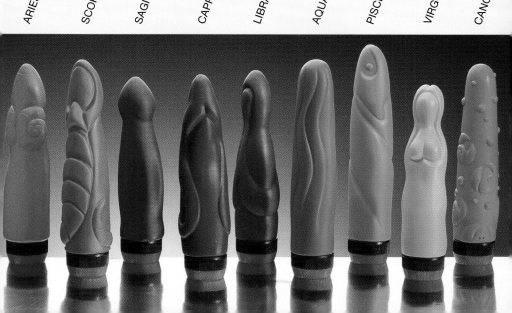

for her | for him | for couples | the bottom line

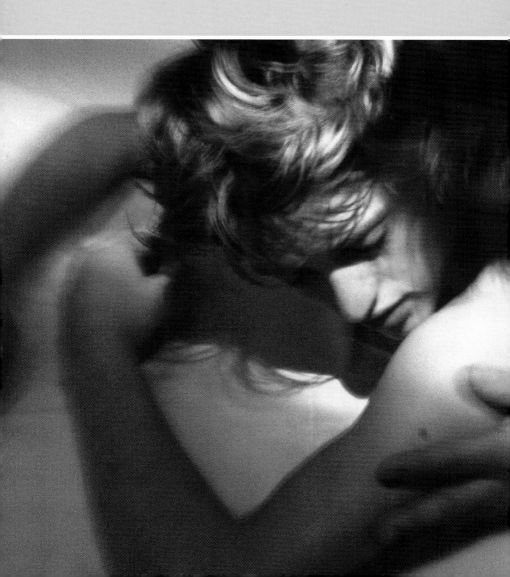

personal playmates

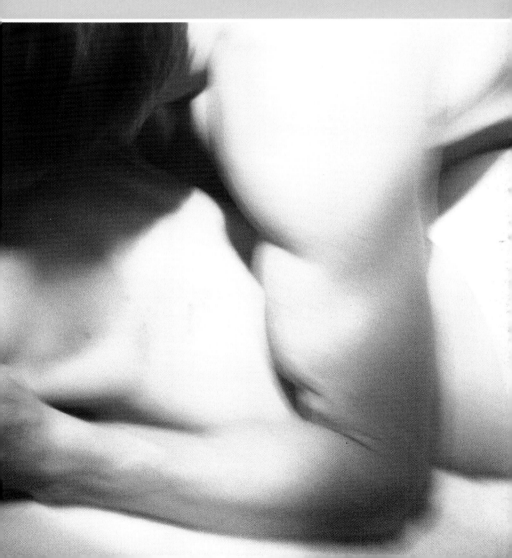

for her

Vibrators are the most popular sex toys for women, and for good reason: they are good value, versatile, portable, and powerful—whether used solo or with a partner.

The humble vibrator, or "vibe" as it is affectionately known, is an innocent, vibrating plaything that can offer sexual pleasure to anyone who chooses to use it. You can enjoy one at home alone, or as an added stimulant with a partner. After all, taking matters into our own hands is often the best way to find out what is good for us. Only then can we begin to coach our lovers, too.

it's a matter of taste
Purpose, shape, size, and color are entirely up to you, but do bear in mind that different vibrators and dildos do different "jobs" (see following pages). As for what your vibrator is made of, it's still a personal choice, but if you are allergic to latex or other plastics you should opt for one made of a material that is safe for you.

> "'Where should one use perfume?' a young woman asked. 'Wherever one wants to be kissed,' I said."
>
> COCO CHANEL

picking your playmate
Choosing a vibrator or a non-vibrating dildo can be quite a challenge. Traditional ones tend to be penis-shaped and quite realistic, particularly the silicone ones. Others come in all shapes and sizes and look nothing like the male member at all. The main aspects to keep in mind when buying one are purpose, shape, power source, vibration intensity, and noise level.

powerful stuff
It's important to discover whether you prefer a vibrator with internal batteries, one with a separate battery pack, or a plug-in model. Also, consider whether you want to be able to adjust the intensity of the vibrations you receive as you play. If so, choose one with a speed adjuster. Toys which have the controls externally are usually the most convenient to use.

good vibes

When you're buying a vibrator:

- switch it on and test it on the tip of your nose to check that its intensity and speed will suit you.

- while you're testing it, think about the noise it makes: is it too loud or harsh-sounding?

- check it carefully for any surface damage or roughness that could harm you when you use it on delicate parts of your body.

- make sure you're happy with its shape, size, and color, and its feel and smell.

- if you're planning on using it in the bath or shower, then always make sure it's a waterproof model.

less purr, more grrr

Don't be afraid to take into account the all-important noise level of your vibrator, too, when making your purchase. Do you really want your friends and neighbors knowing what you're up to? But don't worry—modern technology means that many new vibrators on the market are much quieter and more discreet than in the past.

secret of success

Once you've got your new playmate home, the key to getting the most out of it is simply to experiment in every area to determine what you find the most erotic.

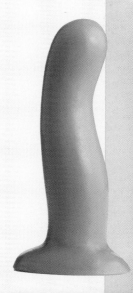

slimline vibes

Slim, smooth, and cigar-shaped, slimline vibrators are effective to use both on the clitoris as well as in the vagina.

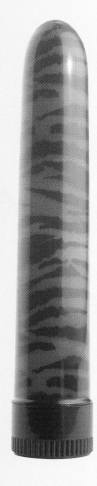

Tiger Temptress

7 inches (17.8 cm) long | hard plastic | internal batteries

Britt's test drive

"I had never used a vibrator before, but this was a really fun product to use. The bright color and modern design initially drew me to it as it made me giggle and relax. It was exciting to play with myself using such a gorgeous toy. The plastic was quite cold to start with, which made it difficult for me to let go and fully enjoy myself, but once I got warmed up there was no stopping me. I enjoyed having no one else to think about but me (and my clitoris) for a change. I found it worked best when I used it with a lubricant, and the sensations varied depending on the depth and angle of penetration. For me, the best effects came with the vibrator about three-quarters of the way in with the base pressed against the back wall of my vagina. A big part of the pleasure was seeing the vibrator in action, too."

sexiness: *grrrrr!*
value: *you won't regret getting this little pet!*
sound effect: *noisy but exciting*

according to ANNE

Slimline vibes are a great toy for first-time vibe users or for those who want maximum sexual stimulation without deep penetration. Their cool, sophisticated look adds visual stimulus, too!

tips for use

Start off by rubbing your toy on various sensitive parts of your body to experiment with the different intensities of vibration. Take your time reaching your clitoris if you are looking for prolonged stimulation—once you get there, your orgasm might be only seconds behind! On a more technical note, make sure that your batteries are the type recommended by the vibrator's manufacturer. With some models, using high-powered batteries can harm the motor.

with a partner
Seductively dart the vibrator along, and in an out of, each other's thighs, then run it along one another's genitals.

spoilt for choice

GRAPE-SCENTED VIBE: this intoxicating toy is 7 inches (17.8 cm) long and sensually scented with the springtime aroma of grapes.

LOVE DOME: this red 7.5 inch (19 cm) vibe has an interesting secret: every time you take it out of its stand you can hear the saucy message you or your lover has recorded!

WATER WAND: a pretty little vibe: 7 inches (17.8 cm) long and aquamarine.

realistic vibes

Unlike the cigar-shaped slimline vibrators, these vibes look more like the real thing. They also feel more realistic, thanks to the use of materials such as jelly, silicone, and luxurious Cyberskin.

Ribbed Red Ruby Jewel

6 inches (15 cm) long | jelly | internal batteries

Helen's test drive

"For me, this vibrator was the ideal length, shape, and girth, close to a good version of the real thing. It was generally firm, with a nice soft surface. To start with, I tried inserting it slowly and deeply while standing, then took the same action while I sat backward on a chair and balanced the toy on the seat. But I found it most enjoyable when I used it lying on my back on the bed. I experimented with the remote control, to vary the vibration speed, but while the highest setting was not unpleasant, it didn't add much value. I eventually brought myself to a lovely climax by stroking my clitoris while moving the vibrator in and out, and I loved the fact that I was controlling the action. The next time I tried it I used a lubricant—a definite improvement. Overall, a pretty good substitute for the real thing!"

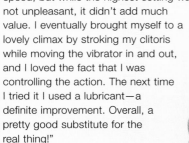

sexiness: *it's getting hot in here*
value: *pricy, but nice*
sound: *wouldn't hear it under the sheets*

according to ANNE

These toys have a sexy look, a sexy feel, and a choice of realistic skin tones or bright, non-threatening colors, such as reds, purples, and greens. Most women find them much better than the smooth, slimline type for penetrative stimulation.

tips for use

A good vibrator is a wonderful aid to satisfying masturbation. Take your time and explore different ways of using it on and around your clitoris, at different depths and angles inside your vagina, and with different styles and rates of thrusting. For extra stimulation, you could fantasize while you play with your tireless toy or use it while you watch an erotic videotape or read a raunchy book.

with a partner
When you're with your partner, don't forget that he'll get a real buzz from the feel of the vibrator on his penis. He'll also get turned on by using the vibrator on you, and by watching your reactions when you use it.

spoilt for choice

RANDY ROD: a curved and determined 8 inch (20.3 cm) black vibrator, elegantly veined and with a proud head. A beautiful piece of work.

THUNDERBIRD: this well developed, firm vibrator is 8 inches (20.3 cm) long, and has a realistic look complete with veins. This vibe has the batteries inside and adjustable speed.

BABY THUNDERBIRD: at 6 inches (15 cm) long, this vibrator is a more modest version of the Thunderbird. Batteries inside, adjustable speed.

EIGHT INCH REALISTIC: 8 inches (20.3 cm) long, pink skin-colored, waterproof and realistic (*very* realistic—even features a foreskin). Batteries inside, adjustable speed.

g-spot heaven

For really intense pleasure, try a small vibrator specially designed to stimulate your G-spot. This type of vibrator has an angled head that you can press against your hidden hotspot for maximum arousal.

Lil' Hotty

5.5 inches (14 cm) | jelly | separate batteries

Gordana's test drive

"I was pleasantly surprised by the gentle texture of this toy and its soft, non–threatening color. When I first used it, I found its sound and the strength of the vibrations a little strange, but I soon got used to them. I started by putting it flat against my clitoris, which felt very nice. Then I inserted it into my vagina with the curved bit pointing up. It didn't do much on its own, but when I fingered my clitoris at the same time it helped me orgasm three times within five minutes—and the orgasms were much stronger than normal! I think that if I used it like this with a partner stimulating other parts of my body, the sensation would be much stronger and I would probably lose myself entirely (still planning to try this!). I also found the curved part of the vibrator was good to use on my nipples, too—it worked wonders!"

sexiness: *swoonsome*
value: *cheap thrills*
sound effect: *murmurer*

according to ANNE

These little vibrators are easier to use for G-spot stimulation than the straight models. The effect can be sublime, but don't worry if they do nothing for you. Not every woman has a G-spot, and having one doesn't guarantee an orgasm.

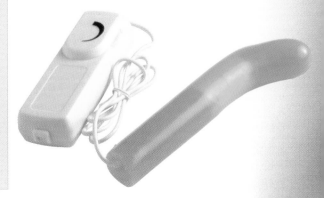

tips for use

Try using one of these vibes to stroke your G-spot with a constant, firm pressure, or vary the stimulation by slowly increasing and decreasing the pressure. It's a good idea to empty your bladder before you start, because sometimes an orgasm triggered by the G-spot can start by feeling like an irresistible urge to pee. If you know your bladder is empty, you won't be distracted by the mistaken impression that you're going to wet yourself. Even so, some women find that the orgasm is accompanied by a gush of fluid from the vagina—female ejaculation! Don't worry, it's not urine. It's a watery liquid that comes from glands called the Skene's glands.

spoilt for choice

NATURAL CONTOURS: about 4 inches (10.2 cm) of beautiful modern design with a subtle, smooth plastic finish. Classy.

FRITZ: this snake-shaped little number, about 6 inches (15.2 cm) long, is perfectly designed to hit the spot.

THE G-SPOT VIBRATOR: this is 7.5 inches (19 cm) of smooth vibrating pink plastic with an angled tip. Does what it says on the package.

TECHNO FLEX: 7.5 inches (19 cm) long, this is a two-speed, egg-shaped vibrator on a flexible shaft. Ideal for getting straight to the point.

JELLY G VIBE: a 6.7 inch (17 cm) pale purple jelly vibe, curved to reach your G-spot.

G SMOOTH: 7 inches (17.8 cm) of pure pleasure! Never fails to deliver the goods.

clitoral stimulus

These little vibrating and flicking toys are designed specifically to tickle your clitoris. Most have a remote control and deliver precisely focused and effective stimulation. Lie back and enjoy!

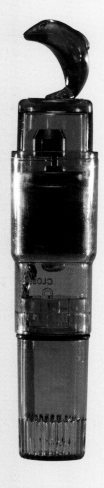

Dolphin Delight

2.8 inches (7 cm) long (4.3 cm) wide | jelly | internal batteries

Claudia's test drive

"This cute little clit-stimulating dolphin flips about at the end of a blue battery compartment/handle. I tried using it while lying on my back and when kneeling, and I liked its strong vibrations. Its soft nose was good for stimulating my clitoris and exciting when I used it on my nipples, but it wasn't very effective when I tried it inside my vagina. However, I liked its harmless appearance—I could leave it lying around the house and nobody would know what it was!"

sexiness: *so stimulating!*
value: *so good!*
sound effect: *so quiet!*

according to ANNE

For most women, effective clitoral stimulation is one of the most reliable routes to an earth-shaking orgasm. With these little gadgets, you can deliver an intense, focused stimulation to drive yourself wild with pleasure.

tips for use

These little vibes are designed to work on your clitoris, but don't let that restrict you. Try delaying the gratification by using one first on your shoulders then gradually working your way down your body. Move it onto your nipples, your belly button, the ever-sensitive bikini line, the inside of your thighs, and finally—as a long-awaited reward—your eager clitoris.

A neat little trick is to switch it to full power and partially insert the vibe into your vagina. Then squeeze your thighs together to feel the vibrations spreading right through your legs and into your whole body.

Cyber Flicker

3 inches (7.6 cm) long | Cyberskin | separate battery pack

Sandi's test drive

"An unusual and surprising shape for a sex toy. I rather like the fact that it's not phallic, so it doesn't feel like some kind of desperate substitute for the real thing, just a way of having a lot of innocent fun! The funky purple color appealed to me, and I absolutely loved the texture. I also loved the delicate sensation it created as it twitched against my clitoris. I tried this while lying on my back, while sitting up, and while lying with my back to my boyfriend with him kissing my neck. Just as I was about to climax, he'd turn the speed down then suddenly turn it up again for great results!"

sexiness: *obscene!*
value: *bargain*
sound effect: *subtle*

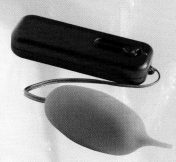

spoilt for choice

PUSSY PLEASER: this little vibrating toy is a soft pink jelly cup with little feelers inside, wrapped around a powerful vibrating bullet. Use it on your clitoris or on your nipples. (And yes, it lives up to its name!)

THE TONGUE: this naughty toy sticks out its tongue at you—then vibrates! Use the separate controller to set the speed, then lie back and let The Tongue give you a good talking to.

double whammy

These vibes pay special attention to your clitoris, brushing across it with arousingly regular movements as the vibrator pulsates inside you.

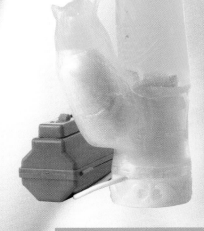

Double Whammy

7.5 inches (19 cm) long; shaft 4.7 inches (12 cm); clit stimulator 3.7 inches (9.4 cm) | jelly | separate battery pack | long nose on clit stim

Rachel's test drive

"Our first impression of this toy was that it was a bit odd. The vaginal bit looked like a sphinx and the clitoral bit looked like a platypus. But when I put the Double Whammy on the bed and switched it on, it came to life and started bending toward me—very endearing! I gave my boyfriend the control, lay back, and let him take over. To start with, he switched on the "sphinx" and slipped it inside me. It didn't have much effect, but things changed when he turned on the "platypus." After guiding his hands to get the toy at the right angle, I was soon close to a powerful orgasm. My vagina muscles actually squeezed the "sphinx" so hard that it stopped being effective, so my boyfriend switched it off and let the "platypus" finish the job. It did so very quickly and I had an intense orgasm, which was quickly followed by a couple more!"

sexiness: *orgasmic (literally!)*
value: *animal magic*
sound: *noisy but interesting*

according to ANNE

An ordinary vibe will either stimulate your vagina or your clitoris—but not both at the same time. This type gives you the choice of vaginal or clitoral stimulation, or both at once. Choose whichever suits your mood and turns you on the most.

spoilt for choice

THE SWAN: 6.7 inches
(17 cm) of soft, pearly-white
plastic with a determined
little clit stimulator on one
side. Heavenly.

LUMINOUS VIBE: 6.5 inches
(16.5 cm) long and made out of
soft, luminous green jelly. This is a well-
equipped vibe with a vibrating shaft, a
beaver-shaped clit stim, and an anal
attachment—it leaves no zone un-probed.

OSAKI BEAVER: this yellow jelly vibe is
6.3 inches (16 cm) and features a
very busy beaver-shaped clit
stimulator. The vibe has an
interestingly arousing twisting
motion. There are two
separate motors, one for the
vibe and one for the clit-stim.

tips for use

With a dual-action vibe like
the Double Whammy, it pays
to experiment a little to find
out what it can do for you.
Try it at different speeds,
starting at the slowest and
gradually increasing to the
maximum—if you can take it!
Also, vary the angle of the clit
stim for different sensations
and levels of stimulation.
Work it at different speeds
over the tip of your clit, on
the sides, at the base, and on
the area around it.

with a partner
When you've mastered your
new toy, teach your partner
how to use it on you in the
way you like best.

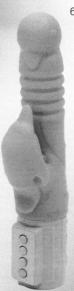

randy rabbits

Used for simultaneous vaginal and clitoral stimulation, these rabbits' movements combine up-and-down and swirling actions to provide exciting changes of sensation.

Jessica Rabbit

4.3 inches (11 cm) long | jelly | separate battery pack | moving internal beads

Kim's test drive

"My first impressions of this toy were not very good. The cartoon-like appearance, slightly rubbery smell, and drab brown control box were not very sexy. But my initial feelings of nervousness, curiosity, and embarrassment soon changed to feeling thrilled and delighted. The variety of motions gave an extra element of surprise, playing with the variable vibe speed was very effective, and the rotation felt sensational. But the effect of the rabbit ears on my clitoris was the best part! The total effect brought me to climax very quickly. When my partner used it on me he enjoyed giving me such pleasure and seeing the smile on my face. However, this toy could be intimidating for a man who isn't confident and might worry that he was becoming redundant —because Jessica Rabbit gives all the satisfaction a good partner can, apart from the hugs and kisses!"

sexiness: *run rabbit, run*
value: *buy—now!*
sound: *varied, but relatively quiet*

according to ANNE

The cute little bunny ears on these toys are a great way to get a solo orgasm or to warm yourself up for sex with your partner. Tickle your clitoris with them at various speeds and you'll soon be wet and waiting for him with great anticipation!

As with other dual-action vibrators, whether you are using a rabbit alone or with a partner, it's best to start off slowly and use the controls to build up the speed. To vary the stimulation you receive you can adjust the pressure of the rabbit ears on your clit—try using the toy with the ears just brushing against your clitoris with a feather-like touch. Experiment with all the different combinations of speed, pressure, and angle to see what you like best, and let your partner know your preferences.

Remember to keep a spare pack of batteries in case the ones in your toy run out mid-action—that would never do when you're having such fun!

spoilt for choice

MINI-JESSICA: this little fun-bunny is 4.9 inches (12.4 cm) long, made of soft blue jelly with bumps on the shaft, a rabbit-shaped clit stimulator, and internal batteries.

WATERPROOF JESSICA: Soft, dark purple jelly, 7 inches (17.8 cm) long. Features a large head and a rabbit-shaped clit stimulator.

THE RAMPANT RABBIT: this yummy bunny is 7 inches (17.8 cm) long, made of pink and red jelly, and has internal batteries. It features a clit-stim and a rotating shaft filled with sensual beads.

glitter vibes

You can use these versatile vibes for a hot evening alone or to brighten up your foreplay when you're with your partner. Their soft feel and warm, glittery colors make them perfect for all the glamour pussies out there.

Shagasaurus

7 inches (17.8 cm) long | jelly | internal batteries | rubber tail

Jackie's test drive

"This is a fun toy, with soft little fins on its back and a little rubber tail for anal stimulation. I liked its color and transparency, and I wouldn't be embarrassed to show it to a close friend. When I looked at the Shagasaurus for the first time, I smiled at the thought of using it. I don't have a partner at the moment, so I used it on my own, lying on my back on the bed. I liked the feel of it inside me, and the feel of the rubber tail on my anus, but I liked it even better when I turned it around so that the tail was on my clitoris. I think it works best when you use it with lots of lubricant (especially on the fins) and at full power! I will definitely be using it again—and soon."

sexiness: *horny*
value: *good value*
sound effect: *noisy, but it's so good it didn't matter!*

according to ANNE

These vibes are a good idea—they combine a realistic size and a (fairly) realistic shape with friendly, fun colors. This makes them a good choice for women who might feel embarrassed by some of the other styles now on the market.

Promise

7.5 inches (19 cm) long | jelly | internal batteries

Ivana's test drive

"This vibrator looks as though it's trying to disguise itself as a kid's toy, but it's definitely only for grown-ups. It's a good size, with a soft and yielding surface, and it's also surprisingly bendable. My boyfriend and I were intrigued at the thought of trying it out, and we took it in turns to use it on me. I lay on my back with him lying on his side next to me. I didn't find it at all embarrassing to use, and it felt much more realistic than I had expected it to. I liked it most when we used it for clitoral stimulation. It seemed to work best like this, as an added extra to foreplay, and it certainly helped me get aroused more quickly—which my boyfriend loved!"

sexiness: *very promising*
value: *complete bargain*
sound effect: *chatterbox*

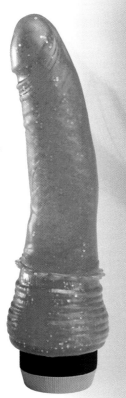

strap-on-vibes

These battery-powered clitoral stimulators come complete with elasticated straps to hold them comfortably in place. Just strap them on, hit the switch, and enjoy the ride!

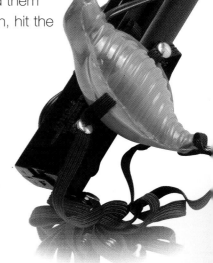

Mini Hummer

3.3 inches (8.4 cm) long, 1.4 inches (3.6 cm) wide | firm jelly | separate battery pack

Anita's test drive

"I was amused by the hummingbird shape of the toy, but I liked the idea of its pecking beak! Although the straps were a little hard to get into, and to adjust or secure, the effort was well worth it in the end because of the amazingly constant pressure that the clitoral stimulator provided. It's not possible for a finger or tongue to apply such pressure, so this was a rare treat. The vibrations sent great muscular waves of pleasure through my whole genital area. When I used it lying on my front, the pressure of the vibrations was increased, much to my delight. But it was also great when I simply held it against myself while sitting, standing, or lying on my back. What's great with this toy is that you have the choice of either directing it by hand or going for the completely hands-free option!"

sexiness: *gives interesting tingles*
value: *worth every cent*
sound effect: *hums discreetly*

according to ANNE

These strap-on toys don't need to be big, because they focus all their effect on your clit for maximum stimulation with minimum effort. Small, discreet, and very easy to use, these tiny vibes can give you a real buzz!

tips for use

Try using some lubricant on your hummingbird for a slightly softer vibrating sensation.

If you are feeling adventurous, you might want to wear a subtle strap-on like the Mini Hummer under your clothes when you go out! Think of the fun you could have at a dinner party—as long as the music is loud enough!

Use the sliding action of the control to vary the speed gradually at first, until you get used to it. Then really go for it with dramatic contrasts in vibe intensity, going ultra-slow one second, and top speed the next. After all that, you'll never be able to look at a hummingbird in the same way!

spoilt for choice

VENUS PENIS: this soft, violet-colored vibrating butterfly has a penis of 6.5 inches (16.5 cm) on its back and elastic straps. It has a separate battery compartment and speed controller. Perfect for hands-free fun.

SWEETHEART VIBE: a firm pink plastic vibrating heart with soft spikes. It is held in place by a black garter belt.

HEART THROB: a small, vibrating purple heart held in place by a sexy black lace garter. It measures 1.6 x 1.4 inches (4 x 3.6 cm) and has a separate speed controller and battery compartment.

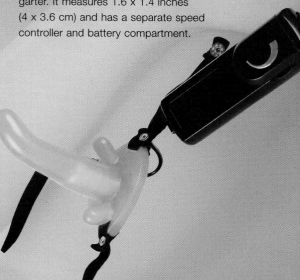

mini magic

Small but perfectly formed, these dinky little vibes can provide surprisingly strong sensations. Slip one into your purse or pocket and have fun wherever you go!

Pop masseur

3 inches (7.6 cm) long | plastic | internal watch batteries

Jenny's test drive

"The first time I tried it, I lay on my back, twisted it up a little way like a lipstick, and used it on my clitoris and the area around it—it felt gorgeous! Then I twisted it up farther and tried closing my thighs now and again while I used it. This spread the sensations through my whole pelvic area and right down my legs, and it made me feel almost out of control with pleasure! I loved using it on my own, but it was such a turn-on it made me want something more than my fingers to penetrate me. So it was even better when I used it on my clitoris and my nipples while my partner was inside me!"

sexiness: *lip-smackingly good*
value: *buy it!* sound effect: *hums*

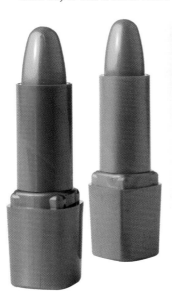

according to ANNE

To get the best out of these little toys, explore the range of different sensations you can get when you use them on different parts of your body. Vary the angle and the pressure or add a little lubrication to provide some extra sensuality.

Finger Fukuoko

3.3 inches (8.4 cm) long, 1.4 inches (3.6 cm)
diameter | firm jelly | separate battery pack

Jasna's test drive

"We started off by practicing with it on
'neutral' parts of each other, such as our
bellies, shoulders, and even noses, to get
used to using it. It felt soft and arousing,
and, once we'd got the hang of it, we took
turns using it on each other's nipples and
genitals—it was a lovely way to spice up
our foreplay, and it soon led to some really
hot sex! We both found it exciting and sexy
to use, and it's certainly a genuine
pleasure-enhancer!"

sexiness: *great name—great toy*
value: *worth its weight in gold*
sound effect: *murmurer*

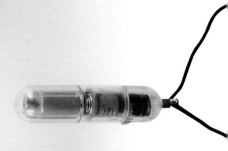

spoilt for choice

WRIST ROCKET: 2.6 inches (6.6 cm) long,
made of purple plastic with a wrist strap to
stop it from flying off.

MICRO DOLPHIN: this is a cute, dolphin-
shaped plastic vibrator. It's 4 inches
(10.2 cm) long, and waterproof.

LOVE TRINKET: this vibrator is a 4 inch
(10.2 cm) treasure of pearl-colored plastic,
with a separate battery compartment.

FINGER TINGLER: keep your digits busy
with this vibrating finger extension which
can be used for both him and her. This one
is 2.6 inches (6.6 cm), cordless, and made
of white plastic.

VIBRATING FINGER: this 3 inch (7.6 cm)
purple vibrator has a spiky, waterproof,
transparent purple sleeve. Sometimes it's
very rude to point!

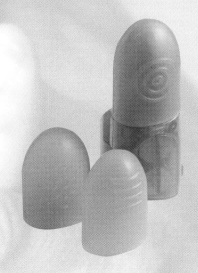

dildo delights

Although vibrators are now more popular, many women still have a lot of fun with non-vibrating dildos. They are made in an amazing array of colors, shapes, and sizes to please their users.

Pink Honey's

6.7 inches (17 cm) long, 1.7 inches (4.3 cm) wide | silicone

Natalie's test drive

"I have to admit that I usually like big boys, but this toy was more than a little intimidating to start with! But the funky pink color made it slightly more friendly and I liked the warm, velvety feel of it. The first time I tried it on my own, I made the mistake of using it before I was wet and it was simply too big to go in. But after a little self-play and a bit of additional lube, I was able to slip it in with no trouble. Now that I'm used to using it, I have to admit that it's very pleasant having something so 'filling' inside me, and I like the smooth, slippery feeling when I move it in and out. I also like rubbing it against my G-spot and nuzzling it against my clit. Sometimes I even double the pleasure by sliding it in and out with one hand while using a small vibrator in the other for extra clitoral stimulation—if my boyfriend isn't around to do it for me!"

sexiness: *filling*
value: *great value*

according to ANNE

Dildos are the simplest sex toys, but in skilled hands they can be very effective. For best results and to avoid discomfort, either use a lot of lubrication or get yourself really excited and wet before trying to insert one.

tips for use

When you're buying a dildo, you'll find that most sex toy stores carry a wide choice of styles. The straight, smooth ones are easy to use and are often a good option if you've never tried a dildo before. The curved shapes can make it easier to reach your G-spot, and while the ridged and knobbly versions can give extra stimulation, you'll probably need to keep them really well lubricated to avoid discomfort. If you're not sure whether to buy a dildo or a vibrator, you could try a vibrating dildo. This is a dildo with a small vibrator that you can insert into its base for extra stimulation.

Width is also an important factor to consider when you're buying a dildo. Don't choose one that's too wide—you'll never be able to use it comfortably.

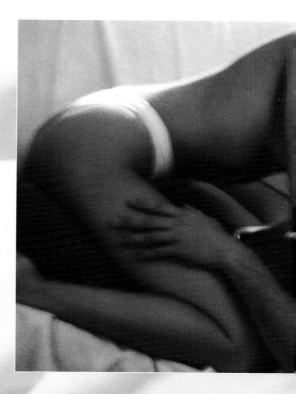

spoilt for choice

GIRLYLUV 1: this is a firm, ribbed dildo, 4.3 inches (11 cm) long in royal blue silicone and with a romantic, heart-shaped base. You'll luv a bit of it.

BUZZ 1: a multi-talented silicone dildo with a small vibe that you can slip into its base to make it vibrate. Available in purple, blue, or black, the Buzz 1 is 6 inches (15 cm) long and 1.25 inches (3.2 cm) wide.

WAVY G: a smooth, S-shaped silicone dildo, ideal for G-spot or prostate stimulation. Wavy G is a very generous 5.5 inches (14 cm) long and 1.5 inches (3.8 cm) wide.

dildos with a difference

Some dildos are straight and smooth, some are curved and knobbly, and some are realistic penis shapes. But others could pass for ornaments on your bedside table…

Cactus Tickler
6.3 inches (16 cm) | silicone | clitoral stimulator

Jenny's test drive
"This glittery dildo made me laugh when I first saw it. I wondered just how comfortable its knobbly texture would be, especially as I am not used to having 'foreign objects' inside me. I needed masses of lube when using it alone, but none at all, much to my surprise, when using it with my partner. He inserted it while I was lying on my back, and, although it initially felt like there were three of us in the bed, I soon rather enjoyed it being there. I liked the fact that it warmed quickly to my body temperature, which made the dildo feel quite natural. The sensation of the knobbly shaft and clitoral stimulator rubbing against me on the outside was great, but I didn't even feel the knobbly texture on the inside! It only took me about ten minutes to have a mini-orgasm, which is pretty impressive for me! It even left me with a warm 'afterglow' sensation, just like the real thing. Next time, I want to try the real thing up my back passage while I do the same thing as before with this—that should be great fun!"

sexiness: *lovely*
value: *well worth it*

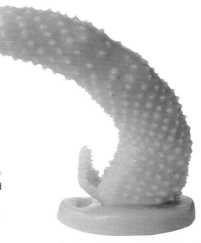

according to ANNE

These dildos look more like novelties than serious sex toys, but they are effective as well as attractive. Their unusual textures and shapes provide interesting sensations for both your vagina and your clitoris.

tips for use

Unlike vibrators, which are intended for external stimulation, dildos are meant to be used for penetration and thrusting. In this respect they simulate intercourse, except that you are in complete control.

Use your imagination when you play with your dildo—relax, fantasize, and vary the strokes; don't just stick to one repetitive motion. Try different rates of thrusting, and alter the angle and depth of penetration to give a constantly changing effect. With a little practice, you will be able to control how quickly you reach orgasm, and have as many orgasms as you can handle! And for a really unusual sensation, try chilling your dildo in the fridge before use.

spoilt for choice

K.I.S.S.: a red silicone dildo, 6 inches (15.2 cm) long and 2.2 inches (5.6 cm) wide. You won't forget your first K.I.S.S.!

TOTEM: this green/brown silicone dildo is 6.3 inches (16 cm) long and has a raised pattern for extra sensation. Quite a pole.

DOLPHIN: a pretty dolphin-shaped silicone dildo that is 6 inches (15.2 cm) long and 1.4 inches (3.6 cm) wide, so it's not for those who like to feel filled.

for him

Why let the girls have all the fun? Boy's sex toys are a growing industry, and you can get all sorts of gadgets and gizmos to help get you up and keep you going, and enjoy yourself more along the way!

Men can have a lot of fun with some of the sex toys designed primarily for women—try using a small vibrator on the head or shaft of your penis, on your testicles or perineum, or around and inside your anus. If that whets your appetite, how about a vibrating sleeve for solo pleasure, a cock ring to keep you up, or a pump to give you an erection to brag about?

sleeve up and down your penis. If you don't like the vibes, you could always opt for one of the many non-vibrating versions. These aid masturbation by copying the feel of a vagina or a mouth around your penis.

swelling with pride
When you get an erection, the spongy erectile tissues in your penis fill with

> "I'm such a good lover because I practice a lot on my own."
>
> WOODY ALLEN

getting a buzz
Give your wrist a rest with a vibrating masturbation sleeve that does most of the work for you. A vibrating sleeve is basically a snug-fitting tube made of jelly or silicone. Using plenty of lube, you slip your penis into it. When you switch it on, a small vibrator sends waves of pleasure through your penis and testicles, bringing you to an effortless climax. You can intensify the effect by sliding the

blood to make it swell and stiffen. A cock ring fits tightly around the base of your penis to make sure the blood stays in and keeps your erection big and firm. The pressure of the ring also helps to delay ejaculation and makes your climaxes feel more powerful and satisfying. The most basic cock rings are simply stretchy rings of plastic or rubber. For added pleasure, the more elaborate designs have moldings or attachments

getting started

A lot of men like the idea of using sex toys like these but are reluctant to try them. This is often because they feel guilty about masturbation, or because they think that using a cock ring or a pump makes them look inadequate. But masturbation is both natural and harmless, as well as being an ideal (and enjoyable!) way to explore your body and improve your sexual stamina. Also, there's no shame in wanting to improve your erection or make it last longer. You'll enjoy it when you masturbate, and both you and your partner will appreciate the difference when you make love!

Don't be too proud to experiment with using toys to enhance your lovemaking—there's absolutely nothing wrong with using a toy to make sex more fun.

that can be used to stimulate either your testicles or your partner's clitoris—or even both!

pump up the volume

A penis pump creates suction that draws blood into your penis to give you a bigger and harder erection than you'd normally get. It doesn't have a permanently enlarging effect, alas, but most men enjoy the sensation of using it and find that the temporary difference is pleasingly obvious.

backdoor man

The prostate gland is often called "the male G-spot." It produces one of the main constituents of semen, and, during orgasm, muscles around it contract to help pump the semen out through the penis. Stimulating the prostate with a finger—or better still a prostate massager—can trigger effects ranging from intense pleasure to sensational orgasms!

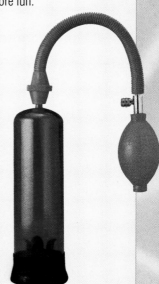

vibe sleeves

These battery-powered vibes for men have soft latex or plastic sleeves, often shaped like mouths or vaginas. They fit snugly around the penis to deliver their arousing vibrations.

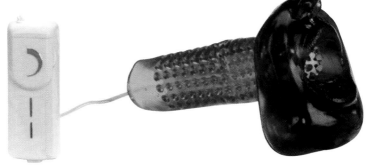

Emerald Lips

7 inches (17.8 cm) long | jelly | separate battery pack | speed controller

Peter's test drive

"The first time I tried this toy I was seated and in a semi-aroused state, and although I put plenty of lube on the 'mouth' and inside the sleeve I had trouble putting it on. The mouth is not very flexible and I couldn't quite get my penis inside it. I thought I might fit into it more easily if I switched the vibrator on, so I tried again with it switched on at a low speed, but that didn't work either, so I gave up. Next time I made sure I was fully aroused before I tried it, and used a great deal of lubrication both on the toy and on my penis. That was much more successful! Although it was a tight fit, I could quite easily move the toy up and down with my hand to add a thrusting effect to the vibrations. That was very satisfying and I came quickly."

sexiness: *voracious*
value: *a sound choice, sir*
sound effect: *eats with its mouth full*

according to ANNE

Vibe sleeves are no substitute for the real thing, but they are great for solo pleasure. And instead of just going for a quick climax, why not use them to practice controlling your ejaculation? That's a fun way to improve your sexual performance!

tips for use

These toys are designed to expand so they can fit penises of all sizes but still grip them firmly. Because of this firm grip, you might find them difficult to get into if your penis is only partly erect. To avoid discomfort, make sure you are fully aroused before you use one.

You should also use plenty of lubrication with these toys—to make them easier to put on, to make the feeling more realistic, and to prevent discomfort. Silicone-based lubes can actually damage silicone toys, and petroleum-based lubes will damage latex, so only use the type of lube recommended by the toy's maker. Also, don't forget to keep them scrupulously clean, and always use a condom if you share a toy with a friend.

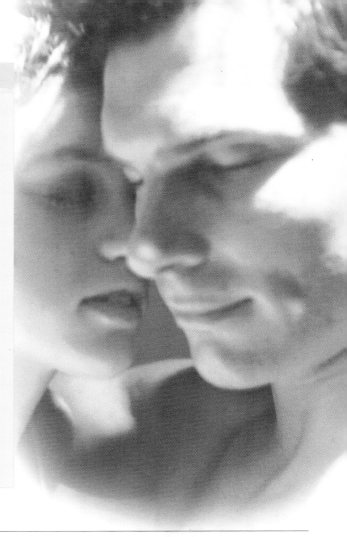

spoilt for choice

POWER STROKE: a soft sleeve with a contoured interior and a mouth-shaped opening enclosed in a transparent purple casing. The action comes from a ring of beads that moves up and down your penis, so the power soon goes straight to your head.

FUTUROTIC EMBRACE: a vibe sleeve with a noduled interior and "tentacles" around the mouth to tickle your testicles.

ECSTASY: this vibrator is molded into the shape of a partly open mouth. As well as vibrating, the toy contains a very talkative tongue that massages your penis.

FLESHLIGHT: this popular non-vibrating sleeve has flashlight-shaped casing with a soft, sensuous lining. A very illuminating experience.

cock rings

Cock rings grip around the base of your penis to keep you harder for longer and make your climaxes more powerful. Some also have clitoral stimulators to give your partner extra pleasure.

Spiky Cock Ring
plastic | spikes

Seb's test drive
"I certainly felt that it kept me hard, both during intercourse and after I climaxed. An unexpected bonus was that I couldn't feel it when it was on—I had expected to feel a tightness or even discomfort. You have to be a bit careful when you put it on or take it off, or it can catch in your pubic hairs. My partner thought it looked funny (like some kind of space insect), but the spikes did the trick for her, although she would have preferred it to be made of a softer material. Overall, we both found the effect pretty amazing!"

sexiness: *throbbing*
value: *so cheap, yet so good!*

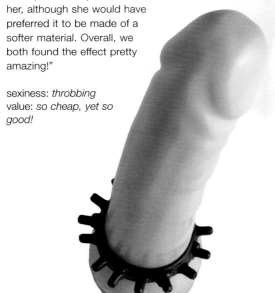

according to ANNE

If you've never used a cock ring before, your best choice is an adjustable one that you can experiment with to find the amount of constriction that suits you best. An added benefit of these is that they're quick and easy to remove.

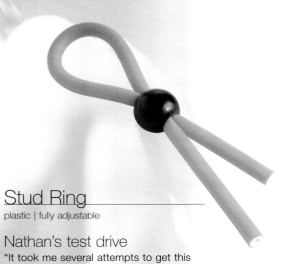

tips for use

Cock rings work by stopping blood from draining back out of your erect, blood-filled penis. You can either slip the cock ring around the base of your penis, in front of your testicles, or place it even lower down so that it is behind your testicles.

For safety, never wear a cock ring for more than about twenty minutes at a time, and take it off immediately if it starts to hurt. You should never use a cock ring if you have circulation or nerve problems, if you are diabetic, or if you are taking any form of anticoagulant or blood-thinning medication, including aspirin.

Stud Ring
plastic | fully adjustable

Nathan's test drive
"It took me several attempts to get this adjusted enough to have any real effect—I was a little fearful of over-tightening it and hurting or damaging myself. But when I finally got it right, I was delighted by the firm and lasting erection it gave me and the way it made orgasms feel more intense and gratifying."

sexiness: *gripping*
value: *lets you take control*

spoilt for choice

ZORRO: a cock ring for master swordsmen, consisting of a fully adjustable soft leather strap with a quick-release mechanism.

POWER: this stretchy silicone ring contains smooth, spherical magnetic beads that massage both you and your partner during lovemaking. *Power!!!*

FULL POWER: this is a set of three stretchy silicone rings of different sizes.

You could even wear one on your penis and another around your testicles. *Even more power!!!*

DOUBLE HELIX: a joined pair of flexible rings, one for your penis, one for your testicles. See, science can be fun.

LOVE LIPS: a soft silicone ring shaped like a pair of luscious red lips. Stretches to fit any size, but holds effectively.

other enjoyment

Try boosting the power of your erection with a penis pump, or use a nice long prostate massager to stimulate your prostate gland for a more intense orgasm.

Big Cock Pump
8 inches (20.3 cm) long | plastic | squeeze bulb | sachet of lube

Justin's test drive
"The pump couldn't have been easier to use—you lube the opening, slip your penis in and squeeze away with the bulb until your penis is rock-hard. My penis didn't get dramatically bigger, but both me and my girlfriend agreed it was noticeably larger and harder than usual, which was easily enough to make the effort worthwhile! We both thought it made our lovemaking more exciting and satisfying, but the best part was when she suggested using it to get me hard again after I had climaxed. It worked like a dream, and now she enjoys 'pumping me back up again' when I've gone flat so that we can carry on again as often as we like!"

sexiness: *insatiable*
value: *big + cock = buy it*

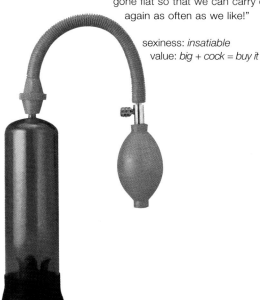

according to ANNE

If you have trouble getting a good, firm erection, try using a pump to make you hard and use a cock ring to help you stay that way. Show your partner how to operate the pump and fit the cock ring so you can make the preparation part of your foreplay!

Black Corker
10 inches (25.4 cm) long | lucite

Tony's test drive
"Stimulating my own prostate was a new and exciting experience for me. The long shaft is easy to handle and I found it easy to reach my prostate with it. The thin tip at the end of the toy worked wonderfully. I could use it to apply steady pressure, or jam it in and out for a lovely, intense feeling. I can't wait to try it out with a partner!"

sexiness: *thrilling*
value: *your prostate will thank you*

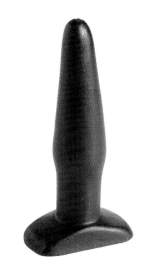

Three Extra Inches
10 inches (25.4 cm) long | lucite

Nathan's test drive
"This is a condom with an extension on the end. Wearing it made me look like I had undergone a botched penis transplant, because it was a different colour to my real prong. However, I really liked walking about with this on and pointing it at my girlfriend. When we became intimate, I enjoyed pulling it out and putting it back in again while marvelling at its length. My girlfriend loved it when I wore this and now won't let me in bed without it!"

sexiness: *this toy is king*
value: *life-changing*

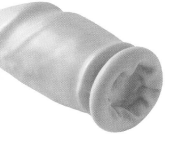

spoilt for choice

TOP GAUGE PUMP: powerful and easy-to-use, with a manly pistol-grip hand pump, a pressure gauge, and a quick-release valve.

POWER SURGE: this is a combined pump and vibrating sleeve. Use the pump action to firm up your erection before sex, or to customize the fit of the sleeve for solo pleasuring. Power is a great aphrodisiac.

for couples

If you like using vibrators and other sex toys with a partner as well as on your own, why not try some toys that are specially designed to be shared?

There are many good reasons for couples—hetero or same-sex—to bring sex toys into their love lives. On the physical level, good sex toys can help both you and your partner to reach new heights of excitement and more powerful and satisfying orgasms. And they can often benefit men whose erections tend to fade, by helping them to stay the course without going limp before they reach the home straight.

is basically a miniature vibe mounted on a cock ring. The ring helps the man to keep a firm erection, while the vibe stimulates his penis and helps his partner to orgasm by working its magic on her clitoris.

the vibe between us

The trouble with sharing an ordinary vibe with your partner is that you have to take turns at enjoying it. Double vibes

> "Personally I know nothing about sex because
> I've always been married."
> ### ZSA ZSA GABOR

On the emotional level, shared sex toys can enhance your feelings of intimacy and trust, and help to put the spice back into your relationship if your lovemaking has become too predictable.

the magic circle

If you're looking for an easy, hands-free way to enjoy the pleasures of a vibe while you're having sex, then a vibrating cock ring could be the answer. This toy

get around this problem by providing you with two different-sized vibes, connected by a cord that carries the battery power to the smaller vibe. Of the two vibes, the larger is usually an ordinary full-sized vibe while the smaller one is slim with an angled tip so that you can use it for G-spot or prostate stimulation, or anywhere else that tickles your (or your partner's) fancy. These toys are extremely versatile—one of you can

getting started

Many people want to bring toys into their sex lives but aren't sure how their partners will react to the idea. If you're in this situation and you don't want to risk a row by raising the subject, try a more gradual approach. Start off by introducing something fun and non-threatening into your lovemaking, such as edible body paints, massage oils, or a furry massage mitt. If these work out, you've shown your partner that using toys is harmless fun, so he or she will be more likely to agree when you suggest using something more adventurous, such as a vibrator or a strap-on dildo. Once they realize how much fun you can both have, they won't be able to keep their hands off you, or the toys!

use both vibes on the other, or you can grab a vibe each and drive each other really wild!

strapping lasses

A strap-on dildo—a dildo fitted into a harness worn around the hips—is a great way for a woman to give her partner hands-free penetration. The strap-on is a popular toy for gay women, but at least a third of strap-ons are bought by straight couples. For these couples, the strap-on allows the woman to have anal sex with her man, and the man can use it if he can't get an erection, or to give his partner something bigger than she's used to. A strap-on can also be useful when playing role-reversal games. With the woman able to act out the part of a man, and vice-versa, the range of fantasies that you can add to your lovemaking is instantly doubled!

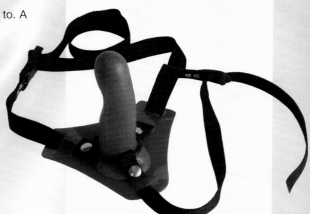

vibrating c-rings

Everyone's a winner when you combine a soft, flexible cock ring with a tiny vibrator. He gets the benefits of the ring, she gets a good clit stim, and you both enjoy the pleasures of a vibrator.

Super Orgasm Sleeve

1.6 inches (4 cm) long | plastic vibe with jelly sleeve | separate battery pack | two speeds

Suzi's test drive

"At first sight, this toy looked hilarious and we wondered if it was a serious sex aid or just a novelty. But it felt nice and soft, so we had no reservations about trying it. My boyfriend put it on his penis and took charge of the remote control (as usual!), and we made love in the missionary position. The soft little spikes around the vibrator stimulated my clitoris in the most sensual way. I had worried it would be rough, but it was nice and gentle. The vibrating feeling went right inside me, making his penis feel like a lovely vibrator. It was a new experience for both of us, and for me it gave exactly the right amount of stimulation in exactly the right places. It didn't really give my boyfriend a great amount of extra sensation, but he did enjoy it. Overall, it was very easy to use (just follow the instructions), and very, very nice."

sexiness: *invigorating*
value: *what else are you going to spend it on?*
sound effect: *hums*

according to ANNE

Clitoral stimulation is a key part of a woman's sexual arousal. The pleasing vibrations of these little toys can often help bring orgasms to women who have difficulty reaching them through vaginal penetration alone.

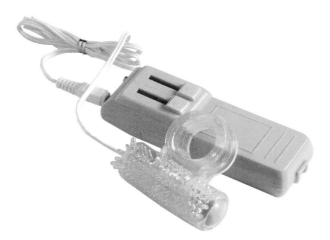

Wittle Wabbit

5.1 inches (4 cm) long | plastic | separate battery pack |

Sally's test drive

"I have never used a sex toy before and was a bit apprehensive about what it would feel like and if I would enjoy it. It took me and my boyfriend a while to work out how to use it. Eventually we found out that when he made love to me wearing it, the rabbit's ears would stimulate my clitoris, while the bit at the end would go into my bottom. I was very embarrassed when we began using this toy and found it quite uncomfortable. However, once I relaxed a bit and got into the swing of things, I started to feel very turned on indeed, with all the new feelings getting more and more intense the longer we went on. By the time we finished, the combination of my boyfriend and the rabbit had me screaming the house down! I am very surprised with how much we both enjoy using this. It is especially effective doggy style."

sexiness: *more!*
value: *looks cheap, feels great!*
sound effect: *who cares??*

tips for use

As well as using these for extra pleasure during intercourse, try using them on each other during foreplay. Work them sensuously all over each other's erogenous zones—anywhere that turns you on, especially the nipples, clitoris, penis, and testicles! To deliver the stimulation more precisely, take the vibe out of the toy and use it on its own.

spoilt for choice

MEGA CLIT TICKLER: a ring with a small vibrator inside a soft jelly sheath with 0.2 inch (0.5 cm) long ticklers. Lives up to its name.

VIBRO RING: a blue jelly ring studded with soft spikes and fitted with a small, remote-controlled vibe. Take control!

ROYAL BLISS: this jelly ring has a remote-controlled vibe and soft ridges. Wear it one way to stimulate her clit, or turn it round to tickle your testicles!

BUNNY C-RING VIBE: a snug-fitting cock ring with a remote-controlled vibe inside a rabbit-shaped sleeve. Lets you buck away merrily.

double the pleasure

A vibe with a separate attachment for clit, G-spot, or anal stimulation can be a good choice if you want to share the fun with a partner. And you can use it on your own, as well!

Double Pleasure Vibe

9 inches (22.9 cm) long and 4.7 inches (12 cm) wide | jelly internal batteries | speed adjuster

Pattie's test drive

"We often use an ordinary vibrator together, so we were intrigued at the thought of using this double one. Our first impressions were that it looked good and had a nice, tactile feel, but initially we found it hard to work out the controls. They were a bit confusing, and when we finally figured them out we were a little disappointed at the small range of settings. But it worked well enough within its limits, although we thought neither part of it vibrated enough. Another drawback for me was that the large vibe was a bit too big for comfortable full insertion, and I found its bumpy surface more annoying than stimulating, but its twisting action was good fun! After a lot of experimentation (which was most enjoyable!) we found that we liked this toy best when we used it on each other during oral sex. That was very nice!"

sexiness: *freaky but fun*
value: *fairly pricy*
sound effect: *mechanical*

according to ANNE

Sharing a vibe is much easier if you use a vibe that is designed to be shared. You can use it on your partner, your partner can use it on you, and you can use it on each other at the same time for truly arousing foreplay.

tips for use

If you are in a settled relationship with your partner and you normally have unprotected sex, you can share a double vibrator without using condoms as long as you use it hygienically. Always clean it thoroughly after you've used it, and be careful not to transfer bacteria from your anus to genitals. It's OK to use the small stimulator first on your genitals and then for anal stimulation, but never the other way around.

spoilt for choice

DOUBLE-ACTION EXCITERS: two small vibrators, one 4.7 inches (12 cm) long, the other 3 inches (7.6 cm) long and both 1.2 inches (3 cm) wide. They are connected to a separate hand-held controller that enables you to adjust the speed of each one individually. The vibrators can be used by you and your partner together, or you can use them on your own if you like burning the candle at both ends.

AUTO EROTICA DOUBLE BULLET: a light-blue, twin-bullet-vibe version of the Auto Erotica (see page 27). It's time to bite the bullet.

DOUBLE STUD: this multi-speed vibe (with a separate control for the clitoral or anal stimulator) should give you plenty to think about. The controls for both are in the base of the main vibe, which features a soft, rotating head and a rotating bead section.

strap-on pleasure

Long a favorite of lesbian couples, the strap-on dildo can also be fun for adventurous heteros if the man is willing to try anal penetration. But remember to use plenty of lube!

Strap-on dildo
6.3 inches (16 cm) long | silicone | you can use the harness with any suitable dildo

Sarah's test drive
"The trickiest part of using this was working out how the harness fitted together—we had to assemble it ourselves with no instructions. Eventually we figured it out, and when I fitted the dildo and put it on I had what we girls apparently long for and harbor bitter envy about not having—a penis. Given that I had a remarkably (for a man) willing partner, I had every opportunity to explore its potential. But, disappointingly, it felt weird because I was just going through the motions with a numb dick. He, however, quite enjoyed it, although he thought it was just a little too big for comfort. The next night we tried him using it on me (vaginally), but I must say that although it felt interestingly large, I far prefer the real thing. Overall, he enjoyed it more than I did."

sexiness: *mmm, delicious, thank you!*
value: *it never wilts!*
sound effect: *strong, silent type*

according to **ANNE**

If you and your partner enjoy using a strap-on dildo, try swapping the dildo for one that can take a small vibrator in its base. If you use it with a harness with no pad behind the dildo, both of you will get the full benefit of the added vibrations.

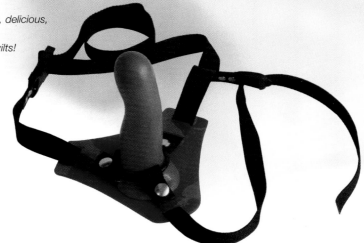

tips for use

You can buy strap-on dildo and harness combinations, or buy a harness and the dildo of your choice. Whichever dildo you choose, it should be harness-compatible—it should have a flange at the base to hold it securely in the O-ring at the front of the harness.

The harnesses available have either one or two straps and are made of nylon or leather. Whether you choose one strap or two is a matter of personal preference, but a single strap allows your partner easy access to your genitals for manual stimulation when you are wearing the harness. Nylon harnesses are cheaper than the leather ones and easier to clean, but they are nowhere near as comfortable. You can also get harnesses that go around your thigh instead of your hips. These can make thrusting easier.

spoilt for choice

SMOOTHIE: a black silicone dildo 6.3 inches (16 cm) long and 1.8 inches (4.6 cm) wide, complete with a luxurious leopard-skin print harness.

OLD DICKIE 2: a pretty pink leather harness with a matching pink silicone dildo 5.1 inches (13 cm) long and 1.6 inches (4 cm) wide.

DIVINING ROD: a silicone double dildo complete with harness. The smaller end is designed to give G-spot stimulation to the woman wearing the harness and the protruding end is 7 inches (17.8 cm) long.

PRIVATE HARNESS: a leather-fronted harness with elastic straps and a sapphire-colored, 7 inch (17.8 cm) jelly dildo. The harness has three different-sized rings, so you can fit it with any size of dildo.

the bottom line

The anus is full of sensitive nerve endings. Anal sex toys, such as vibrators, butt plugs, and beads, stimulate these nerves to heighten sexual arousal and trigger mind-blowing orgasms.

Many people miss out on the joys of anal stimulation because they think it's unhealthy or dangerous, or only for gay men. But unless you have a real distaste for it, it's well worth trying. Done properly, it's extremely intimate, perfectly harmless, wonderfully erotic, and can be a very enjoyable addition to your range of sexual skills, whether you're male or female, straight or gay.

anal vibes

Vibrators for anal stimulation use the same technology and materials as ordinary vibes, but they're specially sized and shaped for anal use. They are slim and often tapered for easy insertion, and many have curved tips for stimulating men's prostate glands. They also have flared bases so that they won't slip out of your hand and disappear inside you.

> "I can remember when the air was clean and sex was dirty."
> GEORGE BURNS

However, to get the most out of using anal toys, you need to remember to always use plenty of lubrication and to make sure that your anal sphincter is completely relaxed before inserting the toy. Good hygiene is also essential—you should use condoms if you are sharing a toy, always clean your toys thoroughly after use, and never use a toy on your genitals (or your partner's) after you have used it anally.

butt plugs

A butt plug is an anal dildo. Some are long, curved, and vaguely penis-shaped, but the usual design is a short, stubby toy with a tapered tip and a recess at the base. The recess allows your anal sphincter to close around the inserted toy. This keeps the toy snugly in place and plugging your butt, leaving your hands free for masturbation, foreplay—or other activities, such as housework!

good vibes

Unlike the vagina, the anus has no natural lubrication of its own. So to avoid pain and damage when you're using anal sex toys, always use plenty of lubrication. With anal toys, the thicker the lube the better—try a good silicone-based lube if you're using latex, plastic, or metal toys, but a water-based lube if your toys are made of silicone.

Along with a well-lubricated toy you need a relaxed anus—if your sphincter is closed tight, you won't be able to get the toy in. Learn to relax your anal area by clenching your buttock muscles tightly for three seconds, then relaxing them. As you relax them, notice how your anal muscles also relax—that's how you want them to feel when you start using your anal toy.

Some types of butt plug have built-in vibes for those who want vibration as well as the gratifying feeling of fullness that comes from using a plug. Another way to get this effect is to use a vibrator on the base of a non-vibrating plug once it's in place. You can also get inflatable plugs that expand after insertion, as well as plugs that vibrate and inflate.

anal beads

Small and easy to use, anal beads are the ideal toy for those new to anal stimulation. Movement is the key to using them. As you slip them in or out one by one, they rhythmically open your anal sphincter then let it contract again. This rippling muscular movement is what creates the unique sensation that anal beads can create.

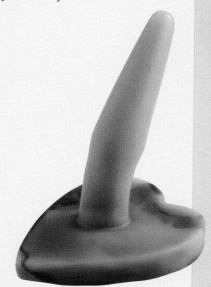

anal vibes

Anal vibes are safe and fun to use. They give you a satisfying sensation of fullness combined with the delicious thrill of waves of vibration spreading through your pelvic region.

Wild Thing
6 inches (15.2 cm) long, 0.6 inch (1.6 cm) wide | plastic | adjustable shape

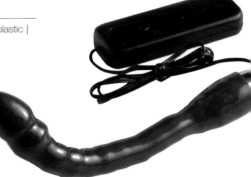

James's test drive
"I used this vibe on my own, while masturbating in bed. My first thoughts were that it was thin and bendy and very solid to the touch, but it would be easy to reach my 'G-spot' with it. I first used in while lying on my back. It was noisy when it bent, and it felt bizarre, uncomfortable, and awkward. But after a while, although it still felt awkward to use, it became increasingly pleasurable. Then I tried it doggy-style, which felt much better, although I would have liked a partner with me to operate the controls. The ribbed surface was pleasant, but turning it around while inserted was a little uncomfortable. It was a good length for pushing in and out, which felt very simulating, though I would have liked it to be a bit thicker. But when I pressed it against my prostate the result was amazing, and pulling it out very quickly when it was set at high speed was just mind-blowing!"

sexiness: *stimulating*
value: *for anal aficionados only*

according to ANNE

Anal vibration is a lovely feeling during both masturbation and foreplay. As a part of foreplay before anal intercourse, it has the added benefit of relaxing the anal sphincter to make penetration easier and more comfortable.

Skinny and Wriggly

9 inches (22.9 cm) long, 0.8 inch (2 cm) wide | plastic | flexible

Tony's test drive

"I'm quite into exploring what my anus has to offer, so I was very up for trying out this little toy. It has a very flexible and smooth tip, and with a bit of lube went up a treat. I used it while masturbating. It actually made things a lot better than I expected and I had a great orgasm in about two minutes. Nice result! Although this looks quite tame, it certainly does the business!"

sexiness: *that tickles!*
value: *a bargain for your butt*

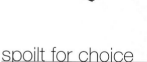

tips for use

Use a vibrator designed specifically for anal use rather than one designed for vaginal stimulation. A proper anal vibrator will be the right size and shape for the job, and it must also have a flared base, or perhaps a retrieval cord, so that you don't lose it. Without these it's all too easy for your toy to slip out of your slippery, well-lubed fingers and disappear up your anus and out of reach. So, make sure that your vibrator definitely includes such physical safeguards!

spoilt for choice

ANAL JELLY VIBE: made out of soft pink jelly, this anal vibrator is a spine-tingling 8 inches (20.3 cm) long.

BEADED ANAL VIBRATOR: this jelly vibe has five prominent beads along the shaft and is 6.7 inches (17 cm) long.

BLUE SUE: a polite little anal vibe just 4.3 inches (11 cm) long. Made of soft blue jelly, it's delicate but effective.

butt plugs

You can use butt plugs in two ways—either work them around inside you for constantly changing stimulation, or just leave them inserted for an arousing feeling of fullness.

The Heart

3.5 inches (8.9 cm) long, 0.9 inch (2.3 cm) wide | silicone | heart-shaped base

Alan's test drive

"This plug was a good size and had a nice smooth surface with a soft, rubbery feel, although I thought the heart-shaped base was a bit sissy—probably a more attractive shape for a female user than for me. However, the thickness of the base did make the toy easy to maneuver during use. I used it lying on my back in bed, and it was easy to position it for entry. It created a great sensation when I started pushing it in, and it felt even better when it was fully inserted. The sensation faded when I just left it in without moving it, but it felt amazing when I started to rotate the angle of the plug and move it in and out. I couldn't really stimulate my prostate with it, but when I twisted it and moved it in and out while masturbating I had an incredible and prolonged orgasm. Would I use it again? Try and stop me! Recommended? Yes!!"

sexiness: *very filling*
value: *your butt needs this plug*

according to ANNE

Using a butt plug will heighten your pleasure and help you to glorious orgasms when you masturbate. And wearing one while you are making love to your partner will add sensuous anal arousal to your genital pleasure.

spoilt for choice

LARGE ASS STUFFER: at 5.5 inches (14 cm) long and 1.6 inches (4 cm) at its widest point, this soft blue jelly plug is a large but comfortable anal accessory.

ASS STUFFER: the Large Ass Stuffer's sassy little 4.5 inch (11.4 cm) brother.

INFLATABLE BUTT PLUG: this is a *serious* butt plug. Once inserted, you can inflate the 4 inch (10.2 cm) long plug to up to twice its original width of 1.4 inches (3.6 cm). It also vibrates.

ACRYLIC BUTT PLUG: 4.5 inches (11.4 cm) long. A sturdy, reliable plug.

PONYGIRL BUTT PLUG: 5 inches (12.7 cm) long and 1 inch (2.5 cm) wide, with a real horsehair tail. Just place firmly into the butt, and hey presto! you have your very own ponygirl.

tips for use

[a]Before you insert your butt plug, use an anal vibe or gently work your finger around inside the entrance to your anus to relax the muscles. Make sure the plug is properly lubricated and insert it slowly, working it around in a gentle circular motion as it slides in.

Remove the plug immediately if you feel pain or discomfort, otherwise you risk damaging the delicate tissues inside your anus.

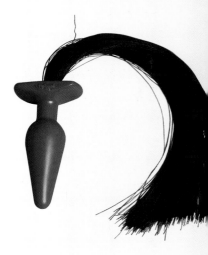

pleasure beads

Enjoy the tantalizing feeling of sliding the beads in and out of your anus, and the sensational, orgasm-boosting effect of pulling them out quickly at the moment you climax!

X10 Beads
11 inches (28 cm) long, 1 inch (2.5 cm) wide | jelly

Tom's test drive
"This long string of tapering beads is quite hard to the touch but also smooth, very flexible, and inviting-looking. The large ring at the end is a very good idea—soft and flexible but easy to hold on to. I used the beads while lying in bed and masturbating. I started off by pushing them all the way in, then slowly pulling them out bead by bead, which was very enjoyable. The sensation changed slightly every time each different-sized bead rippled out. I did this a few more times, before pushing them in one by one, and then pulling them out three or four at a time. When I got near to orgasm, I pushed them all in and pulled them out all at once just before I came. The sensation was unbelievable, I just lost control and had one of the most intense orgasms I've ever had. Incredible!"

sexiness: *fun with fibrillation*
value: *economy*

according to ANNE

If you have never tried anal sex toys before, using beads is a great way to begin. They are small and easy to use, and many newcomers find them much less intimidating than vibes or butt plugs. They are also very arousing!

Jumbo Beads

11 inches (28 cm) long, 3/4 inch (2 cm) wide | jelly

Tina's test drive

"These beads are very wide and very pink—they looked fun, but also a bit scary. I used them with my boyfriend. He enjoyed putting loads of lubricant on them and putting them into my rear end. They felt comfortable but out of the corner of my eye I could see them poking out between my cheeks like a funny pink tail! Anyway, we made love with me on top, while he played with the beads. It gave me some pretty nice feelings and right at the end he pulled them all out. That was great!"

sexiness: *tickly!*
value: *cheap, but still good quality*

tips for use

When you get a set of beads, check them carefully before you use them. Test the connecting cord for weaknesses, to make sure it won't break or start shedding beads when you use it. Then examine each of the beads for raised seams or rough spots. If you find any, carefully smooth them away with a fine nail file or emery board.

When you use your beads—either alone or with a partner—always apply plenty of lubrication. Slowly insert them, one at a time, then pull them out again the same way. As you approach climax, either pull them out slowly to create a rippling crescendo effect, or pull them out quickly to trigger a wonderfully intense orgasm!

spoilt for choice

PURE FLESH ANAL STRING: an 11 inch (28 cm) string of 1 inch (2.5 cm) wide beads made of beige skin-tone Cyberskin. This sophisticated toy features alternate round and oval beads to produce varied sensations and heightened pleasure.

PERFECTION: a stylish string of three pearly pink, 1.25 inch (3.2 cm) vinyl beads.

JELLY PLEASURE BEADS: a pretty 14 inch (36 cm) long string of 0.8 inch (2 cm) pink jelly beads.

JUMBO BEADS: the plastic beads in this 11 inch (28 cm) string increase in size from 0.7 inch (1.8 cm) to a 1 inch (2.5 cm).

all tied up | whipping up a storm

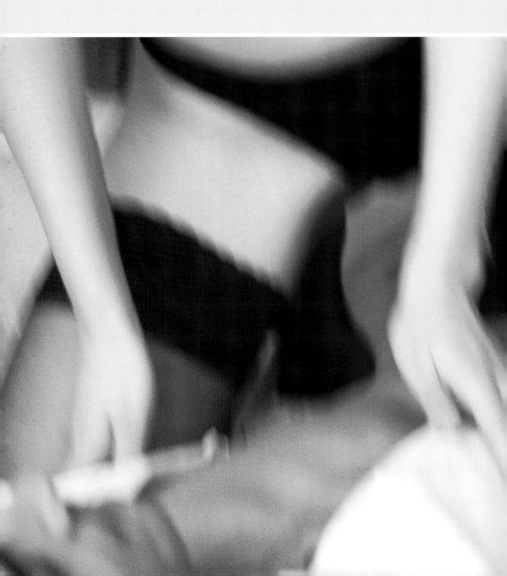

lashings of strappings

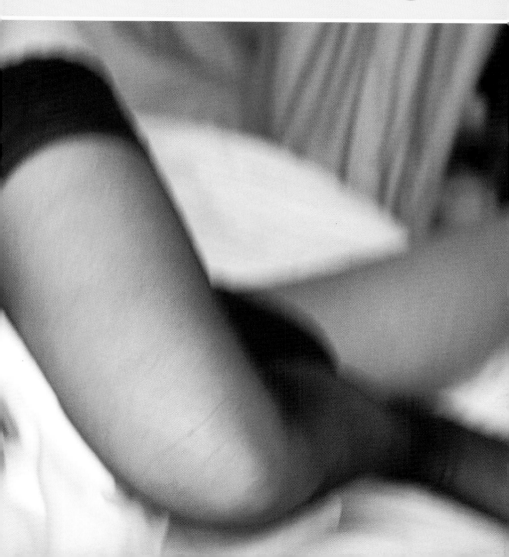

all tied up

Bondage is slowly emerging from its dungeon, and, in a gentler form, infiltrating the bedrooms of countless couples who can get a real turn-on from its erotic potential and its sinful aura of "kinkiness."

A little gentle bondage can broaden your sexual horizons and add some wicked spice to your bedroom bliss. You can use it to act out fantasies of domination and submission or of captivity and rescue, or you can employ your sexual skills to bring your bound and helpless lover to new heights of erotic ecstasy.

If you don't like ropes, or have trouble with knots, try bondage tape instead. Bondage tape is made of PVC, and it's non-adhesive but clings to itself like plastic food wrap. It won't stick to skin or hair, so it's easy to use, and if you smooth it out afterward you can use it over and over again.

"It's been so long since I made love, I can't even remember who gets tied up."

JOAN RIVERS

bound to please
The most obvious way to tie someone up is to use a rope, and the bondage ropes sold by sex stores are soft and supple, making them comfortable and easy to use. You could bind your lover's wrists so that he or she cannot resist your advances, or tie your partner helplessly to the bed with ropes around his or her wrists and ankles before making love to them.

Bondage ties are even easier to use—loops with quick-release Velcro fastenings go over your lover's wrists or ankles, and larger loops attached to them go around the bedpost or any other suitable fixture to provide gentle but effective restraint.

loving cuffs
A fun alternative to rope, tape, or ties are handcuffs—but try not to lose the

good vibes

You don't need to buy ropes, cuffs, or other gear to enjoy bondage. You can improvise by using items such as neckties or scarfs to bind your lover's wrists or ankles, and plastic food wrap as a sexy substitute for bondage tape. But whatever you use—whether store-bought or improvised—there are some basic safety rules that need to be followed.

You should never tie too tightly, use knots you won't be able to undo quickly, or tie anything around someone's neck, however loosely. If you want to use a gag, it must go between the teeth, never over the mouth or nose. Never keep anyone tied up for more than half an hour, leave them on their own, or go to sleep when they are tied up. Before you start, agree on a code word or signal that your lover can use whenever he or she wants to stop.

key! Individual cuffs you can link with connectors or chains are even more versatile and fun. Combine them with a collar and a leash to turn your lover into your personal sex slave!

it's bit nippy in here...

Nipple clamps consist of two clasps connected by a chain. They work by applying a continuous pressure that dramatically increases the nipple's sensitivity, and work equally well on both men and women. They can awaken the erogenous potential of even the most dormant of nipples, and offer an interesting range of sensations—from a gentle squeeze to a tinglingly intense tweak. They can be used solo to enhance masturbation, or with a partner—who just has to give a little tug on your chain to drive you wild! Most clamps are adjustable, so you can control the amount of pressure applied. Remember though, it is recommended you do not wear them for longer than 20 minutes at a time.

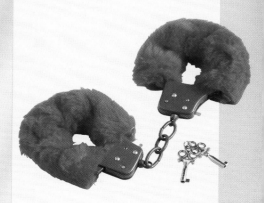

raunchy restraints

Tying your partner up and having them surrender to your will is a great way to add an exciting new dimension to your lovemaking. Combine it with inventive fantasy for a truly memorable experience.

Soft Bondage Rope
23 feet (7 m) long | nylon | includes Japanese Bondage book

Kenny's test drive
"We've never tried bondage before, so we thought we would leave the Japanese stuff described in the book until after we had practiced some simpler things. The first few times we used it, we just tied each others' wrists. This was fun, but it left a lot of unused rope that just got in the way, even when we tied it into a coil. So, we took the plunge and tried some of the Japanese techniques that use up most of the rope. They were simpler than we expected, and, to make it more fun, we pretended that I was some fiendish villain and my partner was my helpless victim. Probably not the artistic approach the Japanese would approve of, but very enjoyable and quite a turn-on for both of us."

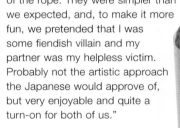
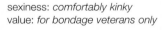

sexiness: *comfortably kinky*
value: *for bondage veterans only*

Tape to Tame
33 feet (10 m) long, 2 inches (5 cm) wide | PVC

Ruth's test drive
"We liked this tape because it was easier to use than ropes (no knots!) and much better than duct tape or parcel tape—it sticks to itself and not to your skin or hair, so it doesn't hurt when you take it off. You can also use it to make a blindfold. Straightening it out again to reuse it was a bit of a pain (you need to be patient), but it's cheaper than buying new tape and you can feel good about recycling it!"

sexiness: *be gentle*
value: *complete bargain*

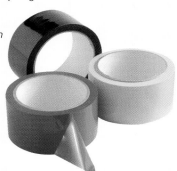

tips for use
Being restrained can be arousing for a number of different reasons—for some people it's the physical sensation of being tied up; for others it's the feeling of delicious helplessness; but for many, one of the biggest thrills is that they get to lie back, do nothing, and be ravished! If you understand exactly why your partner or yourself likes getting tied up, you'll be able to incorporate this knowledge into your fantasies and drive each other completely wild!

Bondage Ties
15 inches (38 cm) long | nylon webbing |
Velcro closures

Dee's test drive
"These were nice and comfortable, as well as fun to use. The Velcro fastening makes them easy to undo, which saved a lot of time when I wanted to get my boyfriend out of them and do something more athletic! It also made the ties more versatile—I could shackle his wrists to the bedposts, to myself, or anywhere else I wanted to park him, while having my way with him!"

sexiness: *naughty*
value: *a luxurious treat*

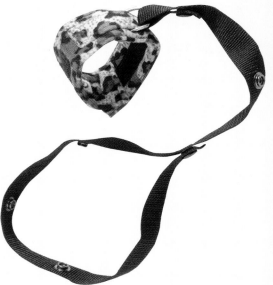

collars and cuffs

Collars and cuffs are among the simplest forms of bondage gear. They're inexpensive and easy to use, but a very effective way of adding erotic restraint to your lovemaking and fantasy play.

Collar and Cuffs

leather | cuff connector

Eileen's test drive

"Our first impression of these was that they were nice to look at but not very erotic—they could have been a fancy-dress item. That's probably because we both usually associate bondage with sinister-looking black leather and plastic gear. When I started wearing them though, we soon forgot about their appearance. Using the cuff connector, my boyfriend could link the cuffs together like handcuffs with my hands in front of me or behind my back, or even link one or both of my wrists to the collar. Also, the metal loops on the cuffs and collar were big enough for a thin rope to go through, so he could tie me to the bed or lead me around like a slave on a leash. And I could do the same to him! All in all, good fun—and we're still finding new games to play with them!"

sexiness: *indecently adaptable*
value: *a bondage bargain*

according to ANNE

Cuffs are extremely versatile bondage toys—you can use them for kinky police fantasies, attaching each other to your bedposts, or even as sexy party accessories. The only limits are your own imaginations!

Leather Cuffs
1.8 inches (4.6 cm) wide | leather, suede, and metal

Helen's test drive
"I like the soft lining of these cuffs, which makes them comfortable to wear even when my boyfriend really fastens them first to make me feel completely restrained. We sometimes use the cuffs with a connector to make them into handcuffs, but mostly we use them with rope through the rings and tie each other to the bed with them. Also, I like wearing one as a bracelet when we go out for the evening!"

sexiness: *luxuriously alluring*
value: *pricy, but good quality*

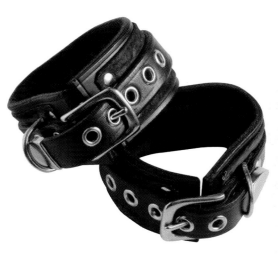

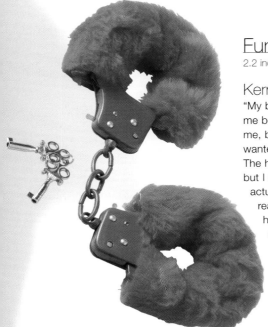

Furry Fantasy
2.2 inches (5.5 cm) inside diameter | metal and fake fur

Kerry's test drive
"My boyfriend got excited at the prospect of me being handcuffed while he made love to me, because he could do anything he wanted, while I could do absolutely nothing. The handcuffs made the foreplay very sexy, but I asked him to take them off before we actually made love—I had gotten really turned on and I didn't want my hands restricted by them when we got really passionate!"

sexiness: *fluffily filthy*
value: *buy them!*

nipple clamps

Both men and women's nipples are a great source of erotic sensations—they can respond exquisitely to licking, kissing, and gentle sucking. But to get the most out of your nipples—clamp them!

Purple Pincher
steel and plastic | adjustable pressure

Gwen's test drive
"I'm into a bit of pain when I'm having sex, so these instantly appealed to me! My boyfriend left them suggestively on the bedside table while we started kissing and touching each other. Pretty soon he decided it was time to clamp me. As soon as he put them on me, my nipples immediately became really hard and I felt an incredible feeling of pain and pleasure mixed together—very intense but very nice! We kept them on while my boyfriend saw to my needs 'down below' and I enjoyed the fact that my whole body became more sensitive. I had to take them off after about 10 minutes though, because it all became a bit too much. I'll definitely use them again, but not too often because I was a little bit sore the next day."

sexiness: *ooh, that smarts!*
value: *classy clamps*

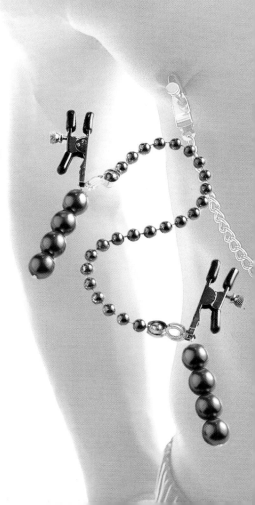

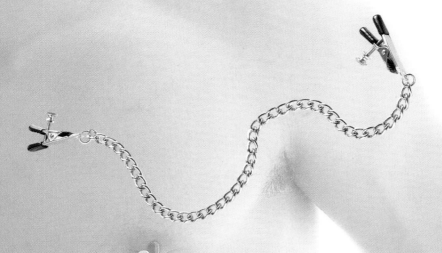

The Nipple Gripper
steel | adjustable pressure

Bryony's test drive
"My boyfriend is completely obsessed with my breasts—he even wrote a poem about them once! As soon as I showed these nipple clamps to him he couldn't wait to put them on me. 'Unfortunately,' I said, 'they're for you!' He was shattered! At first he absolutely refused to wear them, but when I threatened to deny him access to my boobs for a whole month he caved in and gingerly put them on his nips. They have an adjustable 'pain dial' which he set on the easiest level. I enjoyed the look of discomfort on his face and I especially enjoyed giving them a sassy tug. After ten minutes I took them off him and slowly kissed his nipples better—and he loved every minute of it! He said the clamps had made his nipples really sensitive and having them touched felt amazing. So, now I know why men have nipples—it's so they can have clamps put on them!"

sexiness: *intense*
value: *no nipple can escape the Gripper!*

according to ANNE

Many couples in long-term relationships settle into a fairly limited sexual routine after the initial excitement has worn off. Nipple clamps can excite even the most jaded of sexual appetites with some unique combinations of pleasure and pain—keeping your sex life fresh and exciting.

whipping up
a storm

Has your boyfriend been staying out late? Is your girlfriend getting too friendly with the pizza guy? Maybe it's time to flash the whip and deliver a little cautionary discipline!

Sex play involving physical punishment works in a number of enjoyable ways. On the physical level, when you feel pain your brain releases chemicals called endorphins to help reduce it, and these control in the expectation of later reward. And if you're the one handing out the punishment, you get a feeling of power that you might well find very arousing. Such feelings are the basis of

"You don't appreciate a lot of stuff in school until you get older. Little things like being spanked every day by a middle-aged woman: Stuff you pay good money for in later life."

EMO PHILIPS

endorphins give you a brief natural high. Meanwhile, noticeable, but non-damaging impact on the skin makes it much more responsive to gentle stimulation, such as stroking. On the emotional level, letting your lover beat you means surrendering very common sexual fantasies—such as being a wayward lover or a naughty child, or of mistress-and-slave fantasies, which are based on punishment for some pretend misbehavior. You can enhance these with a little spanking or gentle beating.

safety first

Using whips and paddles is harmless fun, provided you follow a few simple safety rules. Firstly, before you use one of these toys on your lover, use it on your own hand so that you can judge how hard you can safely use it. If it's a whip or flail, you should also practice using it on a pillow to learn how to aim it accurately. Never strike your lover anywhere other than on the well-padded parts of the body, such as the buttocks and thighs, and never use a whip on the front of your lover's body or anywhere near the head or face.

whip tease

Unless you and your lover are seriously into pain, whips with single tails are best avoided—they can really hurt and can cause severe damage. The best option is one of the small, soft, multi-tailed whips or flails designed specially for playful sexual stimulation. These are like toy versions of the infamous cat-o'-nine tails. You can use these little whips for teasing and stroking, as well as for gentle lashing. Lightly drag and twirl the ends of the tails over your lover's skin (including nipples and genitals) and see the excitement rising!

hanky spanky

Why not add the power of a paddle or the crispness of a crop to your playful punishment? The wide, flat surface of a paddle spreads the sensation, and some have textured surfaces for sensual stroking. Or—for some aristocratic action—bring out the riding crop!

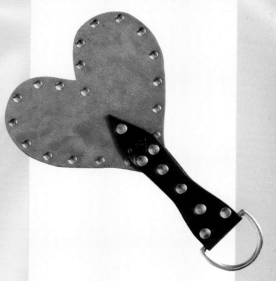

flails and whips

Whip your partner into shape with these stylish chastizers. Use them with a combination of stroking and careful whipping actions to make your partner tingle with delight.

Biz Whip

7 inch (17.8 cm) handle, 18 inch (45.7 cm) strips | black leather strips

Jenni's test drive

"I love whips, cuffs, and really rough sex—I guess I'm a bit of a dominatrix at heart! Unfortunately my present boyfriend is quite inhibited. However, testing this toy was the perfect opportunity for me to 'persuade' him of the merits of a good punishment. I started by leaving the whip on the side of the bed to turn him on. With all its strands and the studded leather handle, it looks extremely dirty! Next, I gave him a full-body massage. After about two minutes I noticed he had a prominent erection. I told him what a naughty boy he was and that he would have to be punished. This made him even more naughty! The Biz Whip gave me good control over the amount of pain inflicted, so I was able to apply just enough correction without him trying to escape from me. I can't wait until he misbehaves again!"

sexiness: *unleash your inner bitch*
value: *a sound investment*

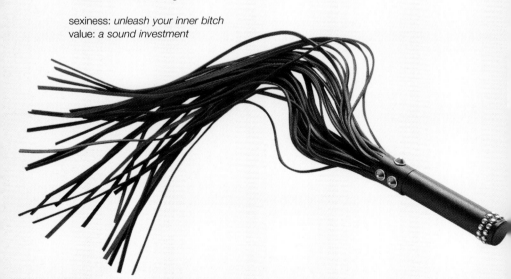

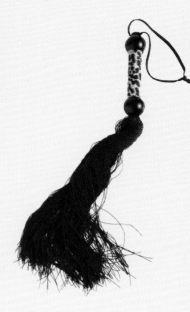

Leopard Lashings

6 inch (15 cm) handle, 18 inch (45.7 cm) tails |
fine rubber tails

Kathryn's test drive

"I started by hitting my partner's butt with the whip
strands while he was fully clothed, then I took his
top off and used the whip as a stroker/tickler on his
chest, shoulders, and back. Next, I laid him on the
bed and pulled off his pants and shorts and then
ran the strands up and down the insides of his legs.
He loved this and it made him moan with pleasure.
We soon swapped places, and it felt amazing to
have so many fine strands hitting me, because they
all struck at different times and spread the
sensation over a wide area. This is one wild toy!"

sexiness: *rampant*
value: *quite pricy*

The Red Rogue

7 inch (17.8 cm) handle, 16 inch (40.6 cm) strips | red leather strips

Gordana's test drive

"The first time we tried it, I was lying on my stomach
and my partner used it on my back. He started off
by stroking me with it, and the most exciting
sensations came when it touched my buttocks.
Then he began hitting me with it, first gently then
more firmly. I loved it, and I was amazed to discover
just how erotic it felt to have my buttocks and lower
back stroked and whipped. I also found it worked
well on my hands and legs, and my partner loved it
when I gently stroked and hit his testicles with it.
That drove him wild!"

sexiness: *sultry*
value: *expensive, but versatile*

according to ANNE

Stroking and light whipping
stimulate the nerve endings
in the skin to produce
highly arousing sensations.
But when you use a whip,
be very careful to avoid
your partner's vulnerable
areas such as the head and
face (especially the eyes).

paddles and crops

For playful slapping, or, if your partner is into pain, for more serious chastisement, nothing beats paddles and crops. Use them for erotic stimulation and in fantasy role-playing that involves punishment.

Heartbeat

7 inches (17.8 cm) long at widest point |
suede, fur, and leather | metal studs

Kay's test drive

"My boyfriend liked me rubbing the furry side on his back, and when I used the velvety side on him, although the studs felt cold at first, he was soon surprised at how much he was enjoying it. Then, when we made love, I beat his butt in time with his thrusts, and he liked that a lot!"

sexiness: *a lovely bit of leather*
value: *expensive, but good quality*

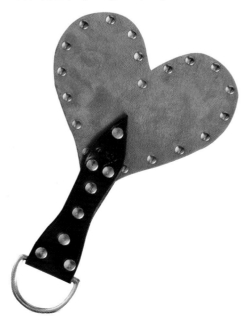

according to ANNE

A little playful spanking can be arousing and fun for both of you, so long as you never hit any harder than your partner wants you to. You can enhance the effect of spanking by alternating it with the contrasting sensations of stroking, caressing, and kissing.

Leather Lashings

6.3 inches (16 cm) and 9 inches (24 cm) long,
plus handles | leather | metal studs

Catherine's test drive

"We tried these out on our hands to find
out how hard to use them, and we liked
the effect and sound of the double layers
of leather. We found that they were best
used with a flicking rather than a slapping
motion, and preferably on fleshy areas
such as the buttocks."

sexiness: *gives them the beating they
deserve!*
value: *discipline is priceless*

Handy Hand

7 inch (17.8 cm) handle, 12 inch (30.5 cm) shaft,
3 inch (7.6 cm) hand| leather hand | wrist strap

Greg's test drive

"We used this in role-playing: chastising each
other for imaginary bad behavior and using it
to beat each other's buttocks. Both of us
enjoyed doing this, but we had to aim
carefully, because the shaft hurts if it hits you.
We also had to be careful not to hit too hard,
because the small hand concentrates the
force of the blow—only hit hard if your partner
really likes pain!"

sexiness: *gets the endorphins going*
value: *great value! buy two!*

rubber lust

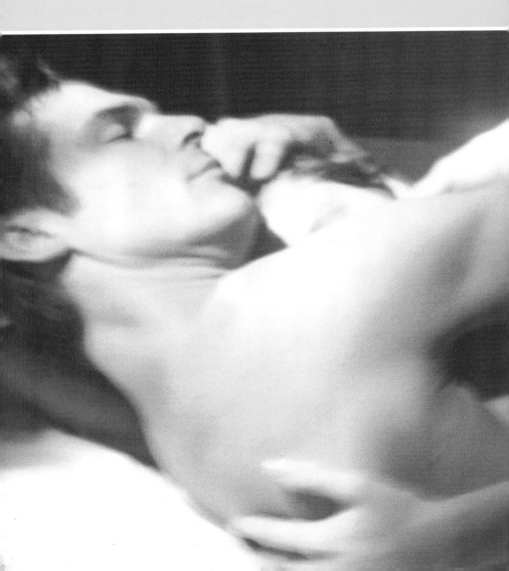

condomania

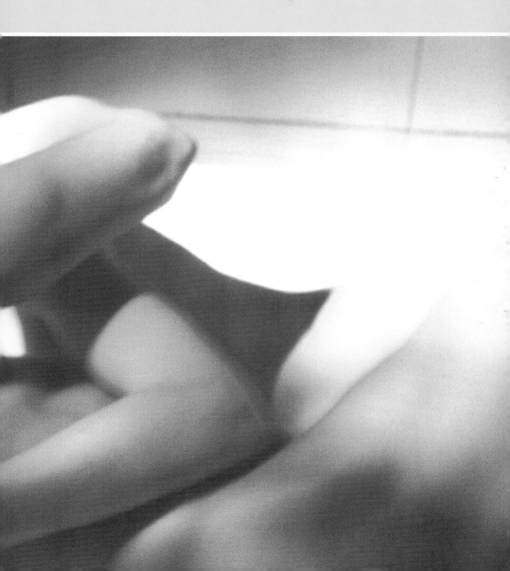

rubber lust

The humble condom has come a long way since the day when it was a sensation-deadening sheath of thick rubber. The modern condom is light, comfortable, and designed for pleasure as well as protection.

Whether you use condoms for contraception or to protect against infection, do yourself and your partner a favor and choose those that combine effectiveness with comfort and sensitivity. With so many different condoms on the market, you should be able to find a style that suits you. Most are safe and reliable, but for peace of mind, it's usually wise to stick to the major brands.

smaller versions if you're a "modestly-built" man or you're worried about finding yourself unsheathed at a crucial moment.

special effects

As if to make up for the lack of flesh-to-flesh contact when you use them, some condoms offer special features for added pleasure. Most often these features are ribs and nubs of extra latex

"In health news, scientists have announced the invention of a woman's condom. The condom works by fitting snugly over the woman's wine glass."

KEVIN NEALON

size matters

A regular-sized condom will stretch to fit any size of penis. A good-quality rubber will stretch enough to fit over your head, and you can inflate some of them with more than a cubic foot of air. But you can get larger styles if you don't like a tight fit (or if you're bragging), and

that are supposed to give women extra stimulation. Some designs work well, while others have little or no effect—but you can have fun finding out which are which! Beware of gimmicky products (including some textured, flavored, and colored styles) that are labeled "for amusement only," or a similar warning.

Remember, those "condoms" are only for fun and you can't rely on them for safety or contraception.

one for the ladies ...

These days, condoms aren't just for the boys. Female condoms—protective sheaths that line the vagina—are just as effective as male condoms, and they give women more control over their own protection. They are made of polyurethane, so unlike latex condoms they won't cause allergic reactions, and they aren't damaged by oil-based lubricants and massage oils, which will ruin a latex condom.

protective headgear

Many people are wary of oral sex, either because they don't like the idea of mouth-to-genital contact or because of the risk of infection from an unfamiliar partner. For safe oral sex, non-lubricated condoms will protect your mouth during fellatio while you can use dental dams to keep you safe when you're giving your lover cunnilingus.

tips for use

If you want a sexy way of putting a condom on your partner, try this method. It's said to be used by Thai prostitutes during sexual massage, and they can do it so proficiently that their clients don't even notice it happening.

While massaging your partner's penis with your hands, put a condom into your mouth. Gently hold the tip between your teeth so that it remains closed and take great care not to perforate it. Then put your mouth over the top of his penis, press the condom onto it with your tongue, and use your massaging hands to roll the condom down the shaft of his penis.

However, always avoid having your mouth make contact with condoms that are lubricated with spermacide, as it tastes extremely unpleasant and can make your mouth feel numb!

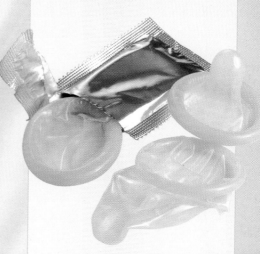

for men

Big ones, small ones, ribbed, or even flavored ones—
whatever your condom needs may be (within reason)
there will be something on the market to meet them.

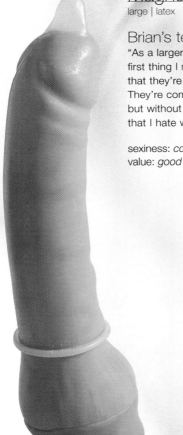

Magnum
large | latex

Brian's test drive
"As a larger-than-average guy, the
first thing I noticed about these is
that they're easy to put on.
They're comfortably close-fitting
but without the feeling of tightness
that I hate with regular rubbers."

sexiness: *comfortable!*
value: *good*

according to ANNE

Don't let putting on a
condom become a passion-
killing distraction—make it
part of your foreplay. When
you're both nearly ready for
intercourse, give him a
gentle genital massage and
finish it by rolling the
condom into place over
his penis.

Pleasure Plus
regular | latex

Jack's test drive
"We didn't expect much from these because we'd tried ribbed condoms before and they were a complete let-down. They did nothing for either of us. But the way the rib-filled section of these condoms slithered around on the head of my penis when we made love was an amazing feeling for both of us. They cost a little more than most condoms, but they're definitely worth the extra money."

sexiness: *slithery!*
value: *costly, but worth it*

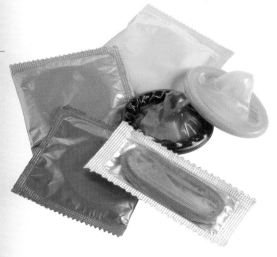

Flavored condoms
regular | latex | flavorings

Ginnie's test drive
"I won't give my man oral sex unless he's wearing a condom, but I find the rubbery taste a bit off-putting, so the idea of flavored condoms was very appealing. However, the reality was a mixed blessing. The mint flavor was nice and the cherry cola was tolerable, and I'd happily use both flavors again. But the chocolate was just horrible!"

sexiness: *tasty!*
value: *complete bargain*

for women

These products help women to enjoy safer sex with male partners, but same-sex couples can also use them when sharing their sex toys or giving each other oral sex.

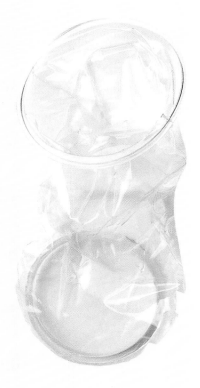

Female condoms

polyurethane | lubricated

Karen's test drive

"After a little practice I was able to get the condom inside me in just a couple of seconds. I've trained my partner to do it so he can slip it in during foreplay, and we don't really notice that it's there during lovemaking. Sometimes it comes out when he withdraws after his climax and sometimes it stays in. Either way, it's quite safe because the open end is outside my body, but you need to take it out soon afterward, or its contents will start to leak out onto the bed. The only drawback we found with it was that the lubricant sometimes seems to get less effective during prolonged lovemaking, so now we always put some extra lube on his penis before we start."

sexiness: *lets you take control*
value: *well worth it*

Polyurethane condoms
regular | polyurethane | lubricated

Mira's test drive
"I don't have a latex allergy but using a latex condom seems to dry me out and make me sore, sometimes even with extra lubrication. No such problems with these condoms, though. Nice and soft, don't need extra lube, and they seem to let us feel each other's body heat better than latex ones do, which is very pleasant."

sexiness: *temperatures will soar*
value: *great alternative to latex*

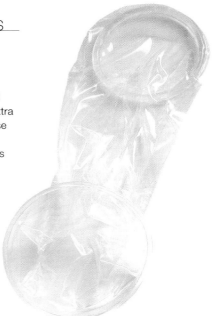

according to ANNE

Nowadays there really is no excuse for not using some kind of barrier to protect yourself against unwanted pregnancy or infection. The female condom gives you more control over your own safety, and polyurethane condoms and dental dams are both effective and non-allergenic.

Dental dams
10 inches (25.4 cm) long, 6 inches (15.2 cm) wide | latex

Cindy's test drive
"My boyfriend is one of those men who find cunnilingus distasteful, so I've been missing out on it since we got together. But getting him to use a dental dam was easier than I expected (perhaps he'd been feeling guilty). Using it was a bit weird at first, but we soon got used to it and now he can give as good as he gets!"

sexiness: *get down to business*
value: *immeasurable*

vibe materials | tubes of lubes | playing it safe

using condoms | looking after your toys

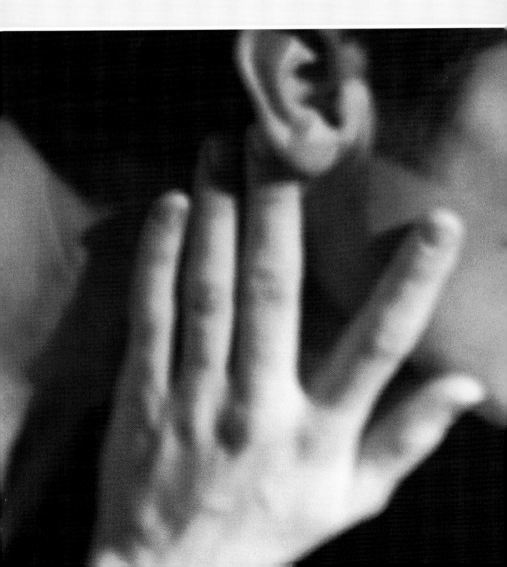

sex
matters

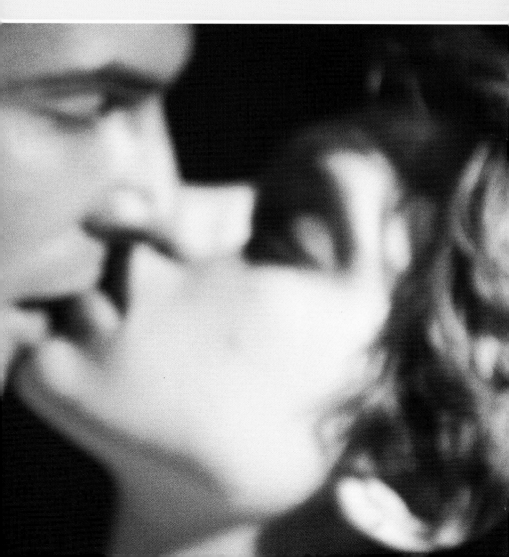

vibe materials

Buying a vibrator or a dildo used to mean choosing between rubber, plastic, and metal. Now you can get your personal playthings in more lifelike and user-friendly materials, like silicone, jelly, and Cyberskin.

All the materials used for making vibes and dildos will do the job, but some do it better than others. As is usually the case, the best ones tend to be the most expensive.

plastic and metal

Vibrators and dildos made of plastic or metal have hard surfaces, usually smooth but sometimes fluted or textured. The hardness of these materials transmits vibrations easily, so plastic and metal vibrators tend to give more intense sensations than those made of softer materials such as latex.

silicone

Silicone is a soft synthetic rubber, naturally smooth with a velvety feel and a relatively non-porous surface. During use, it warms quickly to body temperature and retains its heat, which enhances its lifelike feel. Be careful not to damage a silicone toy with your teeth, nails, or jewelry. Small cuts will spread easily into tears that make the toy unusable. Never use one with a silicone-based lubricant. The two silicones are chemically different, and the lube will ruin the surface of the toy.

jelly

Although less expensive, jelly looks like silicone and has a similarly lifelike feel, but it's not as smooth and flexible and its surface is more porous. Because of this porous surface, it needs careful cleaning with soap and water or a water-based sex-toy cleaner. Avoid using silicone- or oil-based lubricants with jelly because they will damage it.

latex

Latex (rubber) is firmer and more solid than silicone and jelly, but it softens when it gets warm. It's only about half the price of silicone, but it's less flexible and less durable, with a porous surface that's prone to flaking. If you want a vibrator made of latex but you're allergic to the material (or your partner is), always remember to cover it with a new polyurethane condom each time you use it.

cyberskin

The most realistic dildo and vibrator materials are spookily similar to human skin. Sold under various trade names, including Cyberskin, Ultra Skin, and Futurotic, these materials are soft and warm with a smooth and silky texture. This luxury comes at a price, though, as these materials are more expensive than the others. Because they are very porous they need careful cleaning, and you should never share a sex toy made from them without using a condom.

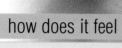

how does it feel

plastic and metal
Hard, cold, and inflexible, but gives intense vibrations; safe to share if wiped clean with alcohol and then water after each use.

silicone
Soft and really lifelike; safe to share if washed with soap and hot water; expensive.

jelly
Soft but not too realistic; a little sticky with a slight plastic smell; only safe to share if used with a condom; expensive.

latex
Firm but still flexible; use a condom to share; costs very little.

cyberskin and ultra skin
Very realistic, but expensive; also very porous, so not safe to share; should be cleaned with a specially formulated cleaning kit.

playing it safe

If you're not sure that your dildo or vibrator is perfectly clean, play it safe and cover it with a new condom each time you use it. And always use a condom if you want to share your dildo or vibrator with a partner.

tubes of lubes

If you want some slinky, sensuous sex, give yourselves a little lube before you make love. Remember, slippery hands make solo sex far smoother and slippery toys feel more sensual.

Good lubrication makes sex wonderfully easy, and results in much more satisfactory penetrative sex. During vaginal intercourse, a woman's natural secretions normally lubricate the contact between penis and vagina. But sometimes this natural lubrication isn't quite enough. For example, if a woman is nervous at the beginning of sex, it may take a while for her vaginal secretions to flow freely, and there are some women who just don't become as lubricated as others. Using a good lube will overcome these problems. Lubricants are helpful when you're using condoms, and they are vital for anal intercourse and the insertion of sex toys.

know your lube

The countless brands of lubricant on the market today are based on either water, oil, or silicone. Most are water-based, which makes them easy to wash off and harmless to the materials used for condoms and sex toys. The only real disadvantage of water-based lubes is that they tend to dry out during use, so you sometimes have to re-apply them.

Oil-based and silicone-based lubes must be used with care, because although they work well as lubricants they can cause problems. Oil-based lubes will damage latex condoms (but not polyurethane ones) as well as latex toys, while silicone-based lubes will ruin silicone toys. In addition, oil and silicone lubes aren't easy to wash out of the vagina, where they can harbor infection. For similar reasons, oily, latex-damaging household products—such as cooking oils, suntan oils, moisturizers, and petroleum jelly—are a bad idea as lubes. And it's always best to keep massage oils and lotions away from latex condoms and toys, unless they are specially formulated to be latex-friendly.

choose your lube

Whatever your lubrication needs, it's essential to use a safe and suitable product, and for most purposes a good water-based lube is the best choice. Some of them, such as Sensilube (Senselle) and Astroglide, are formulated to resemble natural vaginal lubrication in transparency and consistency. Many are available in several versions, such as a light version for greater sensitivity and a thicker one for more substantial lubrication. The thicker water-based lubes are ideal for use during anal sex, as are silicone-based lubes. Then there are entire ranges of lubes that are specially produced for pure fun. These come in wonderful colors and flavors— think Mango, Red Apple, and Wild

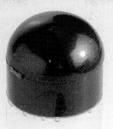

Blueberry—all packaged in brightly colored fun bottles. They are quite harmless if ingested and are, incidentally, sugar-free!

use your lube

Always store your lube somewhere warm, or warm it before you use it, because a cold lube can be a bit of a passion-killer. The best way to apply a lube is to pour or squeeze some into the palm of your hand first, and then smooth it onto (or into) the body part or toy you want to lubricate. Keep some tissues handy so that you can wipe excess lube off your hands after you've applied it. For convenience, you could wash out an empty pump-action soap dispenser and fill it with lube. Then you just need one hand to dispense the lube when you need it.

playing it safe

Unfortunately, sexual activity can sometimes put you at risk of catching a sexually transmitted disease. Practicing low-risk activities and the proper use of condoms will help protect you against infection.

reducing risk

Casual sex—and sex with a new partner at the start of a relationship—carries the risk of infection with any of a large number of sexually transmitted diseases (STDs). These STDs range from thrush and chlamydia, through to syphilis and the most dangerous STD of all HIV, the virus that causes AIDS (acquired immune deficiency syndrome). For examples of activities that carry the risk of transmitting HIV, see the box on the right. All these diseases can be spread by oral, genital, and anal contact and by the exchange of bodily fluids such as semen, vaginal secretions, and blood. The best way to reduce risk is to use condoms during vaginal or anal sex, and condoms or dental dams during oral sex.

feeling safe

While using a condom or dental dam is a cheap and effective way of keeping safe, many people can be reluctant to bring up the subject of safe sex in a casual relationship or a one night stand—even though these are the situations that put you most at risk. It is common to imagine that asking a partner about safe sex may offend them. However, it is essential to get over any embarrassment—not only is it vital for your health, but feeling confident that you are completely safe will eliminate any anxiety during sex. And as everyone knows, anxiety is a big passion killer.

according to ANNE

Penetration need not occur every time a couple have sex. Dry kissing, embracing, stroking, and massage all express closeness eloquently and with minimal risk of infection. Mutual masturbation may be used in the same way, but to be extra safe the active partner should not allow any semen or vaginal fluid to come into contact with his or her fingers, in case there are any cuts, abrasions, or open sores on them.

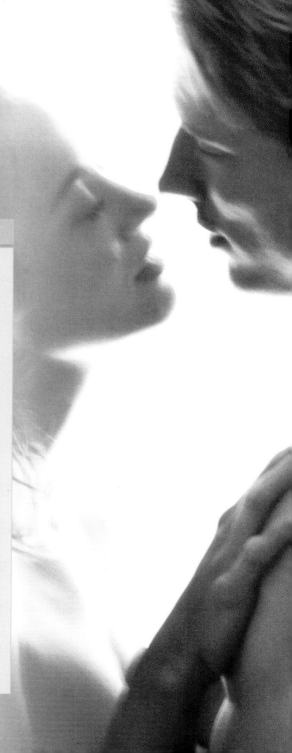

HIV and AIDS

AIDS is caused by a virus called HIV (human immunodeficiency virus). The examples below are ways in which the virus can pass from one person to another

high-risk sex activities
- unprotected vaginal intercourse
- unprotected anal intercourse
- unprotected fellatio, especially to climax
- unprotected cunnilingus
- unprotected anal licking
- sharing penetrative sex aids, such as vibrators or dildos
- inserting fingers or hands into the anus

medium-risk sex activities
- anal intercourse with a condom
- vaginal intercourse with a condom
- lovebites or scratching that breaks the skin
- mouth-to-mouth kissing if either partner has bleeding gums or cold sores
- cunnilingus using a latex barrier
- fellatio using a condom
- anal licking using a latex barrier

using condoms safely

Putting on a condom is easy—but you still need to remember a couple of important points. A condom slipped on incorrectly is worse than useless—it gives you a false sense of security and may result in some very unpleasant surprises at a later date!

using condoms

To help ensure your safety (and your lover's) always use a good-quality condom, never reuse a condom, and never use one after the expiration date printed on the package. When you use a condom, the golden rule is that you should never unroll it before putting it on. To put one on, take it out of its foil wrapper and gently pinch the tip between your thumb and forefinger to squeeze all the air out of it (be careful not to damage it with your fingernails). This is important because if you put the condom on with air in the tip, that air will form a bubble that can burst the condom during vigorous intercourse. And if it does burst you are at risk both of infection and pregnancy. While still pinching the condom, place it on the head of your penis with one hand and unroll it down the shaft with the other.

condom foreplay

A woman can make slipping a condom on her lover's penis a loving, sensual, and erotic action, and turn it into an integral part of lovemaking. She should begin by giving him a gentle massage, and then changing her hand action from massage to gentle masturbation.

Remove the condom carefully from its foil packet, and squeeze out the air by holding the tip between thumb and forefinger, and use slow, sensuous movements to roll it into place. If her partner is not circumcized, she should gently push back his foreskin before unrolling the condom.

talk tactics

Knowing when to raise the issue of using a condom with a new partner is difficult. You may worry that if you broach the subject very early, you are making the assumption that intercourse is definitely going to happen. If you bring up the subject when you are already in bed together, however, it may be too late to take precautions. The best idea is to talk about the issue when you feel sure that you and your partner want to have sex but before you become too intimate.

Your partner may feel relieved that you have broached the subject. If not, point out that using a condom will make you feel safer and better able to relax and enjoy yourself. If your partner resists, you may need to reconsider your relationship. Remind yourself and your partner that condoms are not optional. They are vital.

femidom

These female condoms are an ideal way for women to take control of contraception. They have the advantage over male condoms in that they can be put on before lovemaking begins so as not to inhibit spontaneity. Also, some men find that putting on a condom can make them lose an erection. Although this can be easily cured by putting on the condom as part of foreplay (see left), Femidoms can still provide a great solution.

Femidoms are easy to insert. Like male condoms, they need to be carefully taken out of their packet to avoid tearing with fingernails or jewelry. The Femidom needs to be placed gently on the opening of the vulva, and then slowly inserted by placing a finger into the vagina. It is important to make sure that the bottom rim of the Femidom is completely outside of the body in order to prevent the Femidom from slipping up while you are having intercourse.

looking after your toys

If you take good care of your sex toys you can be confident that they will be clean and safe to use. They will last longer and won't let you down when you most need them!

Proper care and maintenance of your vibrators and other sex toys is essential if you want to keep them clean, safe, and pleasant to use. If you do not keep them clean, they can harbor bacteria that will make them unpleasantly smelly, as well as a source of potentially dangerous infection.

Always clean your toys carefully after you've used them. What you use to clean them with will depend on what they are made of. To clean toys made of Cyberskin or similar materials it's best to use the cleaners specially formulated for them. You can safely clean most other materials with a sex toy cleaner (available from sex toy stores) or simply use alcohol or soapy water. But do remember, when you clean a battery-powered toy, take care not to let water get into the controls or the battery compartment.

To clean a metal or hard plastic toy, wipe it thoroughly with cotton balls lightly soaked in rubbing alcohol, then use a damp washcloth (one that you use

only for your toys) to wipe away the alcohol. Clean latex toys in the same way, but remember that because latex has a porous surface that bacteria can lurk in, it's wise to fit a clean condom to the toy each time you use it. You can clean silicone toys with hot, soapy water (you can even boil them, if they're not battery-powered), but jelly toys are best cleaned simply by wiping them with a damp washcloth—no soap, detergent, or boiling water for these! Remember always to read the instructions that come with the toy because they will tell you the best way to look after it.

storing your toys
Toy storage can be a tricky issue. The best place to keep them is in a drawer close to your bedside so that you have easy access to them when the mood moves you. If you don't want members of your family to find them, it's sensible to stash them in a lockable drawer or box. Another way to hide your sex toys from prying eyes is to keep them in one of the disguised storage containers sold in some sex toy stores. These can take

the form of pillows, fake books, or anything with hidden compartments to tuck your toys into.

Wherever you store your toys, it should be clean and dust-free. When you want use them again, rub them down with oil-free baby wipes to get rid of any dirt they may have picked up during storage. If you're storing battery-powered toys that you don't expect to be using for some time, remove the batteries in case they start to leak and corrode the casings and mechanisms within the toy.

index

suppliers

www.allvibrators.com
tel. (1) 719-532-4103

Ann Summers
www.annsummers.com
tel. (44) 0845-456-2320

www.blowfish.com
tel. (1) 800-325-2569

www.hardtobuy.com

www.lovehoney.co.uk

www.mypleasure.com
tel. (1) 866-697-5327

www.nawtythings.com
tel. (1) 800-779-8077

www.passion8.com

www.sexshop35.co.uk
tel. (44) 0800-018-4137

Sh!
www.sh-womenstore.com
tel. (44) 020-7613-5428

www.takemetobed.co.uk
tel. (44) 01132-94742

www.tickledonline.com
tel. (44) 01273-628725

www.treasuresbysherry.com

acknowledgments

The author and publishers would like to give very special thanks to everyone at Sh! for their help and expertise, Ann Summers for their support and assistance, Pepin Press for the use of their images, as well as Expectations for the whip, and Regulation Ltd for the leather briefs.

Carroll & Brown would also like to thank:
Design Peggy Sadler
Picture Research Sandra Schneider
Production Karol Davies, Nigel Reed
IT Support Paul Stradling

Picture credits
pp8-9 The Pepin Press
P38 www.passion8.com
P45 Ann Summers
P47 top and bottom images
    www.sweetdesire.co.uk
P49 www.blissbox.com
P51 www.sweetdesire.co.uk
P53 top www.blissbox.com, bottom
    www.sweetdesire.co.uk
P55 Ann Summers
P56 Ann Summers
P59 www.blissbox.com
P61 www.blissbox.com
P67 www.sweetdesire.com
P68 www.sexshop365.com
P79 www.blissbox.com
P87 www.blissbox.com